PLEXUS - Treating Vagus Nerve - Practical Guide

Treating Vagus Nerve – Techniques and Remedies in Everyday Life – Practical Guide for Family

A Book written by Loren Allen in collaboration with Dr. Vishen R. Kohler

© Copyright 2022 by Loren Allen - All rights reserved.

The following Book is reproduced below with the goal of providing information that is as accurate and reliable as possible. Regardless, purchasing this Book can be seen as consent to the fact that both the publisher and the author of this book are in no way experts on the topics discussed within and that any recommendations or suggestions that are made herein are for entertainment purposes only. Professionals should be consulted as needed prior to undertaking any of the action endorsed herein.

This declaration is deemed fair and valid by both the American Bar Association and the Committee of Publishers Association and is legally binding throughout the United States.

Furthermore, the transmission, duplication, or reproduction of any of the following work including specific information will be considered an illegal act irrespective of if it is done electronically or in print. This extends to creating a secondary or tertiary copy of the work or a recorded copy and is only allowed with the express written consent from the Publisher. All additional right reserved.

The information in the following pages is broadly considered a truthful and accurate account of facts and as such, any inattention, use, or misuse of the information in question by the reader will render any resulting actions solely under their purview. There are no scenarios in which the publisher or the original author of this work can be in any fashion deemed liable for any hardship or damages that may befall them after undertaking information described herein.

Table Of Contents

Who is the Author	3
Introduction	5
What is the Vagus nerve?	13
Location and Functions of the Vagus nerve	15
The Parasympathetic Nervous System	17
Foods that stimulate the vagus nerve	21
How to Activate the Vagus Nerve	28
Cryotherapy	29
Deep Breathing	43
Gargling	46
Yoga	48
Tai Chi	50
Singing and Chanting	50
Physical Activity	51
Massages	53
Massage guns	54
Acupuncture	57

Chiropractic treatment	58
Cupping	66
Moxibustion	70
Tui na Massage	72
Aromatherapy	73
Sleeping on your right side	77
Coffee enemas	79
Binaural beats	85
Daily Vagus exercises	89
Exercises for Postural defects	91
Exercises for stiff neck	104
Trapezius Exercises	108
Facial Exercises	112
Exercises to increase social engagement.	122
Abdominal Massage	130
Ear Exercises	137
Visceral Massage	142
Neck Massage	143
Breathing immobilization technique	147
Tongue Exercises	148

Foam Roller Exercises	152
Quick Vagus nerve reset.	162
Jaw Massage	165
Foot Massage	171
Sensory Deprivation tank	173
Treating the Vagus Nerve	177
Vagus Nerve Treatment Through Acupuncture	181
Treating the Vagus Nerve Through Mind-Body Therapy	183
Vagus Nerve Toning	184
Conclusion	185

Plexus - Treating Vagus Nerve - Practical Guide

Who is the Author

Loren Allen is dedicated to helping others become their best self and live a happy and healthy life. She loves to write and focuses on topics that can make a real difference in helping others accomplish their goals and dreams. She has made it a habit to continue learning new things so that she can share these insights with the world in a concise and helpful way. Loren was born in 1973 and has earned degrees in Business and English with a minor in Psychology.

She has been very successful in the business world for twenty years and is now moving on to her true passion of being a full-time author.Loren has spent much of her life discovering and implementing self-development strategies. Over time, she has become an expert at the best techniques that can really make a difference for a happier and more fulfilling life.

Her favorite role models are Sheryl Sandburg and Oprah Winfrey. Favorite quotes: "Being confident and believing in your own self-worth is necessary to achieving your potential" - Sheryl Sandburg."My philosophy is that not only are you responsible for your life, but doing the best at this moment puts you in the best place for the next moment." - Oprah Winfrey.Loren loves the outdoors and likes to walk or run every day.

She is dedicated to the practice of yoga and feels that meditation is important to both success and happiness. Her driving passion is to pass on to others the knowledge she has gained to make their lives better.

Introduction

Some people chose to address the organ that was having difficulties rather than looking at the entire system. You may be curious about what a vagus nerve is and what it does. Vagus is derived from Latin and French languages, which mean "wild" and "vagabond." The term "vagus nerve" comes from the idea that it extends from your brainstem to your visceral organs via sensory fibers. It's called "vagus" because it's a stray or roaming nerve that courses along the stomach. Because it is the tenth pair of nerves to emerge from the brain, it is appropriately named the tenth cranial nerve. The vagus nerve collects nerves that run from the gut to the heart and then to the brain. It is the longest cranial nerve and communicates with all of the body's organs. Our bodies are holistic systems that work in unity.

The vagus nerve can be a significant cause of inflammation, arthritis, anxiety, depression, gastrointestinal issues, chronic stress, and other problems if it is not properly regulated. As a result of this research has shown practitioners to treat it in order to avoid putting the entire body through agony. Some healthcare systems focus only on the problem identified at first glance and treat it instead. This may quickly lead to polypharmacy as well as missing the underlying source of the symptoms. Medicine's current approach exhibits this pattern. Medication prescribed by doctors only tackles symptoms and not the root cause of the problem. However, many people don't realize that medication comes with harmful side effects that can lead to polypharmacy. For example, did you know that insomnia or gut health issues could originate from something as profound as the vagus nerve? The vagus nerve is one of several nerves in the body responsible for connecting the brain to other parts of our anatomy, but its importance cannot be understated. The vagus nerve is a primary player in keeping the body ticking. It runs from the brain stem down both sides of the neck, through the chest, and into the belly. In other words: it connects practically all of our critical organs to the brain.

Plus, it's directly related to two areas known for playing roles inalertness and awareness. The vagus nerve has a wide variety of functions--too many to list here! And because it's so important, there are also many ways that you can stimulate it. The vagus nerve is a sensory communication line that informs the brain about what's going on in our bodies, particularly the digestive system; stomach and intestines, lungs and heart, spleen, liver, kidneys, as well as a variety of other nerves involved in everything from conversation to eye contact to facial movements. The vagus nerve not only connects to various organs throughout the body physically but also functions as a messenger through sensory messengers known as chemicals. The vagal nerve terminals have various functions throughout the body, including stimulating the heart's pacemaker and increasing resistance to breathing in the lungs. In addition, they activate smooth muscles in the walls of the stomach and intestines in the alimentary canal, as well as releasing hormones that increase nutrition storage from the pancreas. It is essential for maintaining overall health.

It is a vital component of the parasympathetic nervous system, which is in charge of relaxing organs following the stressful "fight-or-flight" adrenaline reaction to threats.

The vagus nerve is responsible for relaying information from the brain to the internal organs and regulating the body's reaction during periods of rest and relaxation. However, this nerve can become overstimulated, under-stimulated, or damaged. When this happens, it disturbs the messages sent from the brain to the rest of the body. but there are ways you can take care of these instances. The good news is that there are a number of home exercises you can do on a daily basis and foods you may start eating more frequently. This book will assist you with this. We'll also look at the vagus nerve's roles, as well as what irritates and stimulates it. Gargling and cold water therapy may seem like basic, small measures, but they can go a long way in helping to improve your vagus nerve function. If you often find yourself struggling with chronic stress, anxiety, depression or post-traumatic stress, it might be because of issues with your vagus nerve. In this article, we'll teach you breathing techniques that can help stimulate your vagus nerve and promote natural healing. You'll also learn about some common irritants that can impact the health of your vagus nerve. You can assist stimulate the vagus nerve with basic and easy modifications to your lifestyle.

Vagus nerve stimulation is also being studied in various mental illnesses, including epilepsy.

It's also used to treat bowel issues like Crohn's disease and cardiac problems. Such therapy has been labeled a breakthrough in both science and medicine. Taking into account the role of this nerve, it becomes obvious that its impact on the body is significant. Who wouldn't want to cure one-to-many medical issues with basic home exercises that target just one major nerve and can address a wide range of medical issues? I don't believe anyone would say no.

This theory isn't based on wishful thinking or flimsy evidence, in case you were thinking that. Scientists have studied the vagus nerve, which is why the polyvagal theory was created. This has been proved to be a successful approach after many studies and journal articles were published. Although the phrase "the vagus nerve" suggests that a single nerve will be addressed, this is not the case. This refers to a network of nerves. Depending on the disease, this system may assist in natural healing by supporting the body's own healing mechanisms. It helps people become more aware of external and internal stimuli as well as how to deal with them. This book will not have you reciting meaningless words while breathing out your problems, contrary to what you might believe now. This book is designed to give you enough information on the topic in order to now seem vague. The goal of this is to provide you with a clear understanding of your internal system and how modest modifications and adaptations may help you improve your general health, rather than relying on traditional drug therapy. Vagus nerve medicine and healing are approached differently. This approach, unlike traditional medicine, teaches us to avoid and heal sicknesses naturally if they already exist.

Preventing illnesses may help you avoid getting sick in the first place.

Obesity, chronic inflammation, depression, anxiety, seizures, low heart rate anomalies, faintness, and Gastrointestinal problems have all been linked to vagus nerve dysfunction by researchers.

By the end of this book, you'll be able to see just how amazing the human body is and how much control we have over our daily lives when we take a proactive instead of reactive approach. The vagus nerve plays a vital role in many of our bodily functions, even something as simple as saliva production, so don't worry if you're still not entirely sure what it is or what it does! Because a traditional medical method is usually used, few people are aware of this nerve. And if you don't know it exists, how will you care for it? How will you stimulate the nerve if you've been on pills your entire life? Nowadays, more research and journals are being published that shed light on this important section of the body. After reading this, you will understand more about the vagus nerve- how to take care of it and what steps you can now take to ensure its proper function.

What is the Vagus nerve?

There are twelve cranial nerves in the human body, most of which only serve a handful of functions. For example, some govern our sense of sight or hearing, while others control more specific sensations like the sensation of a single finger against our cheek.

However, number ten on this list - the vagus nerve - plays a much larger role and is responsible for numerous function we may not even be aware of; such as the muscles that let us speak or the sensation inside our ear. Cranial nerves are the nerves that connect the brain to various parts of the body, including the head, neck, and thorax.

Sensory information is transmitted to the brain, including details about odors, sights, tastes, and noises. Sensory nerves have sensory capabilities. Other cranial nerves control different muscles' movement as well as certain glands' function. The functions of the brain's motor system are known as motor activities. Some cranial nerves are solely sensory, while others are both sensory and muscular. The vagus nerve is one of these nerves.

According to the Roman numerals assigned to them, the cranial nerves may be classified in three groups: those that originate in the base of the skull (cerebral), those that originate in the middle ear (middle), and those that originate at or above the level of where a human being would have their ears attached (transverse).

The vagus nerve is sometimes referred to as X Cranial Nerve. In the medulla oblongata, it begins. It is located at the very bottom end of the brain, just below where the brain and spinal cord meet. The vagus nerve is made up of two large nerves with long fibers, and these are where the nerves pair. One emanates from the right side of the medulla, whereas the other issues from the left. However, when speaking about the vagus nerve, most people think of it as a single entity without boundaries on either side. These fibers are composed of many tiny cells that distribute information throughout the body. The vagus nerve is responsible for controlling the body's nervous system. It helps the body to relax and digest food properly. The sympathetic nervous system controls the body's fight-or-flight response, while the parasympathetic division helps the body to rest and heal.

Location and Functions of the Vagus nerve

The vagus nerve has two types of sensory functions: somatic and visceral. Somatic components are feelings felt on the skin or in muscles, while visceral sensations are felt in organs. The vagus nerve provides touch information for the skin behind the ear, exterior part of the ear canal, and certain regions of the throat, among other areas. The vagus nerve does a lot more than people realize. Not only does it provide sensation to the voice box, esophagus, lungs, heart, and most of the digestive pathway - it also plays a small role in tongue taste sensation. It dilates the pharynx, larynx, and soft palate; a fleshy region in the rear of the roof of the mouth that stimulates muscles in the heart and lowers resting heart rate. It also aids in the stimulation of involuntary contractions that enable food to pass through the digestive system—going through the esophagus, stomach, and intestines.

The eighth cranial nerve is the longest and most complex in the entire brain. It contains sensory nerves that extend from different parts of a person's body, providing sensation to muscles and glands. A portion of these motor nerves reach up into the brain through the abducens nerve. The main function of this nerve is to send signals to other areas of the body via spinal interneurons. Let us take things step by step, beginning with its origin. This nerve processes touch in your ear and informs you if something has gotten trapped inside it. The vagus nerve controls the muscles of the vocal chords in the throat. This aids individuals in communicating with others vocally. It is also responsible for pharyngeal reflexes and back-of-the-throat motions. Vomiting can be caused by the gag reflex, which is well recognized as causing regurgitation. This reflex frequently helps to prevent objects from getting trapped in the throat and triggering choking. The vagus nerve surrounds the digestive tract, beginning at the esophagus and going all the way down to its termination in the abdomen. The vagus nerve controls peristalsis, or the wave-like muscular movement that food through the intestines.

It aids in digestion, reproduction, and urination by assisting the body in completing tasks that are put off while it is rested.

The vagus nerve, when activated, can slow the heartbeat and reduce blood pressure. The nerve also extends into the lungs, where it aids in breathing regulation. Even the smooth muscle that compresses the bladder when you urinate is controlled by the vagus. It also regulates perspiration. This nerve receives feedback from bases all around the body after sending messages out of the brain. The tips in the brain's vagus nerve help it keep track of all of the organs it goes through. When the vagus nerve isn't under strain, messages are transmitted to the body, slowing heart and breathing rates while also increasing digestion. During periods of stress, control is passed to the sympathetic system, which has an adverse influence.

The Parasympathetic Nervous System

The nervous system is made up of many nerves that help the body to move, react, and detect outside stimuli. The autonomic system has two divisions: the sympathetic and parasympathetic components. Simply put, these are two parts of one larger system. The PSNS starts in the brain and consists of long fibers that connect to certain neurons near the target organ.

This way, once they reach these neurons, PSNS signals only have a short distance to travel before reaching their destination organs. The PSNS can affect various areas such as the eyes, nerves located in the bladder and stomach, trunk muscles, and salivary glands. The purpose of this system is to maintain your fundamental functions. To provide a comparison, the sympathetic nervous system (SNS) increases heart rate. In most cases, a faster heart rate pumps more oxygen-rich blood to the brain and lungs.

This might give you the energy to escape an aggressor or sharpen your senses in another scary situation. The PSNS and SNS are opposites of each other: the former prevents your body from overworking while the latter triggers the fight-or-flight response. Essentially, if you know how the PSNS works, then you also understand how its opposite, the SNS, functions.

The main difference between them is in speed, location, and mode of action.

The vagus nerve, which runs through the neck, is a crucial communication route between the brain and other parts of your body. The cranial nerves are paired nerves that control many actions and emotions in your head and neck.

Every nerve starts in the brain. The 12 cranial nerves are numbered from I to XII, with the first pair of nerves placed at the front of the brain. The oculomotor nerve, which controls the size of the pupils, the facial nerve, which regulates saliva production in the nose and mouth, and the glossopharyngeal nerve that aids parotid gland functioning under the tongue are three prominent cranial nerves. The vagus nerve, numbered X, is another prominent cranial nerve. It's estimated that approximately 75% of the PSNS fibers originate from this one nerve. Scientists have already found that it branches in various organs such as the bladder and sexual organs (among others). Some reflexes of the PSNS are increased salivation and production of enzymes to help with digestion. The tears produced by the lacrimal gland keep your eyes hydrated and help preserve their delicate tissue. During urination, the PSNS (parasympathetic nervous system) causes your bladder to contract so that you can urinate. During digestion, the PSNS is responsible for peristalsis – the movement of food through your intestines and stomach.

It also helps trigger bile production from the liver to aid in fat digestion. Finally, during defecation, the PSNS constricts various sphincters in order to move feces through your digestive system and out of your body.

Your PSNS is a vital component of your body's fundamental activities. When it stops functioning properly, you may experience a variety of physical problems that have a negative influence on your health.

Foods that stimulate the vagus nerve

Many people believe that food is the answer to all of their health problems, but there are a few things you can do to help your vagus nerve function properly. You may select vitamins from naturally occurring foods or go for store-bought ones if you wish to make minor adjustments to your diet.

The vagus nerve may assist the brain and gut by feeding the beneficial gut bacteria with probiotics. The idea is gaining credibility, particularly in the treatment of anxiety and depression.

The vagus nerve serves as a barrier for signals from gut microbiota to the brain. Probiotic strains such as Lactobacillus rhamnosus and Bifidobacterium longum have been found in studies to reduce stress and sadness, while bad bacteria induce anxious behavior. The vagus nerve is responsible for reducing anxiety.

Probiotic-rich foods have been shown to alleviate stress in both human and animal studies. Foods high in Probiotics include cottage cheese, yogurt, kefir, apple cider vinegar with mother, sourdough bread, kombucha, and fermented vegetables like kimchi, sauerkraut ,and pickles.

Lactic acid is a by-product of fermentation and can be found in fermented foods, which are beneficial to organisms. Fermented meals have been shown to impact brain activity. Fermented beverages aid in the formation of signaling molecules that travel through the vagus nerve to the brain, helping to maintain inflammation at bay.

Consuming a diverse array of fruits and vegetables aids in the breakdown of prebiotic fibers, which are necessary for bacteria to create metabolites that benefit brain function. Furthermore, synthesizing neurotransmitters such as serotonin and dopamine is another advantage that bacteria have on brain function.

Prebiotic fibers are found in a variety of whole, natural foods and are beneficial to your gut bacteria. In humans, prebiotics have been shown to lower stress hormone levels. High fiber-rich foods (which tend to be less processed) are also more complex carbohydrates .

Diets high in simple carbohydrates can cause your blood sugar to spike, making you feel more tired after eating. Consistent elimination also helps remove food residues that could potentially accumulate and inflame the colon. This process creates a less ideal environment for organisms that might have harmful effects on the connection between the brain and gut.

Omega-3 fatty acids such as EPA and DHA, which are mostly found in fish, have been linked to improved heart rate variability and vagus nerve activity. Fish consumption and fish oil supplementation have both been shown to improve the nerves, brain, and heart.

Research suggests that omega-3s can improve gut health and reduce the risk of brain disorders in both animals and humans. Bone broth is also a nutrient-rich food that has been shown to aid in healing a leaky gut, alleviate symptoms of arthritis, and improve skin elasticity, hair, and nails.

Bone broth is a liquid made from boiling animal bones and connective tissue. It contains minerals like calcium and magnesium, as well as vitamins A and K2. Bone broth is also a good source of omega 3 and 6 fatty acids, zinc, iron, and selenium.

The connective tissue in bones produces glucosamine and chondroitin, which are effective treatments for joint pain and arthritis. Although you can make your own bone broth, the process might be too time-consuming for some people. Fortunately, there are many good commercially prepared bone broths available from your local grocery store.

Polyphenols, which are plant chemicals absorbed by your stomach flora, are found in cocoa, green tea, olive oil, and coffee. Polyphenols support gut bacteria and may aid cognitive function. Choose dark chocolate with a high percentage; the higher the proportion, the better. To minimize pesticide exposure while drinking organic green tea, choose 100 percent green tea instead of blended varieties.

To guarantee the roots of your beans, select single-origin coffee. To be precise, there is no such thing as a "serotonin pill" or "succussion," but there are supplements that may help boost levels of this neurotransmitter. Tryptophan is an amino acid that, after processing, produces serotonin, a neurotransmitter.

Tryptophan is converted in the intestines to tryptamine, which can help astrocyte cells in the brain and spinal cord control inflammation, potentially enhancing communication between the gut and brain via the vagal messenger system. Spinach, seeds, nuts, bananas, and chicken are some of these meals.

Although choline found in red meat and eggs offer benefits to your health, consuming them in moderation is key. When taken in excess, it can convert to trimethylamine N-oxide (TMAO), which then causes inflammation and cardiovascular problems. To help the vagus nerve control sympathetic vital signs such as heart rate and blood pressure, reducing consumption of certain foods may be necessary.

Some studies have shown that fasting and dietary restriction can activate the vagus nerve. This may be because fasting causes a decrease in metabolism, which the vagus nerve senses as a drop in blood glucose. The vagus nerve also senses when there is less mechanical and chemical stimulation from the gut.

The longer you fast, the more you slow down your metabolism. Increased vagus nerve activity from the liver to the brain appears to lower metabolic rate by increasing vagus nerve stimulation. Fasting has a slew of advantages, ranging from enhanced cognitive function to weight loss to decreased inflammation, so it's worth a try. The nicest thing is that in order to get advantages, you don't have to fast for a long time.

Maintaining healthy eating habits and exercising regularly are the best things you can do to lose weight if you are overweight. I advise that you get some form of exercise every day, and eat a diet rich in vegetables, fruits, nuts, seeds, and legumes like they do in the countries around the Mediterranean Sea.

Refined sugar damages the brain by deranging cellular feedback mechanisms and other communication pathways, as well as disrupting gut mucosal lining inflammation, allowing infections to spread inflammatory signals to the brain. It may help you maintain a healthy brain by altering the types of bacteria in your stomach, which affects the gut-brain axis.

How to Activate the Vagus Nerve

The vagus nerve is integral to maintaining overall wellness, and now it's time to learn how to activate this vital node. The parasympathetic nervous system is activated by increasing vagal tone; meaning, the higher your vagal tone, the quicker your body can recover from stressful situations.

Don't be concerned if your vagal tone is low; you can raise it by stimulating your vagus nerve. It will allow you to more effectively react to the emotional and physical symptoms of your brain and mental illness.

Try the following practices at home to help create a vagal tone:

Exposure to cold water

Cold tubs, or what we commonly know as Jacuzzis, are popular not just in Japan but also in many Northern countries. Here, people take dips in the water to celebrate special occasions during winter or early spring. However, getting used to such frigid showers can be quite a task.

Research has demonstrated that acute cold exposure can stimulate the vagus nerve and cholinergic neurons. Furthermore, repeated exposure to cold water lowers your sympathetic "fight or flight" response while conversely increasing parasympathetic activity through the samevagus nerve pathway.

Utilize cold water for the last 30 seconds of your shower, then work up to longer periods of exposure. Tomate a "hot and cold plunge" by switching between hot and cold water every five minutes. If that's too extreme, start with dipping your face in ice-cold water five times for 20 seconds each.

If you can't bear the thought of taking a cold shower or bath, it's still beneficial. The vagus nerve is activated, which lowers heart rate, increases stomach motility, and boosts the immune system. Do not be scared to go for a walk when it is chilly outside. Toss ice cubes in a Ziplock bag or a towel and press them against your face for an icy facial treatment. The diving reflex is when you plunge into water with hands cupping your face.

Cryotherapy

Someone stroking your skin or the cold wind on your face might provide examples of somatic feelings felt on your skin or muscles. Visceral sensations include bodily changes sensed in the body's organs. You may experience these effects while your entire body is exposed during a comprehensive cryotherapy session.

Cryotherapy, which is also known as "cold therapy," is a therapeutic technique that involves exposing the body to extremely low temperatures for an extended period of time. As a consequence, your body can notify you via the Vagus Nerve that it is too cold, signaling you to lower your stress response and inflammatory cytokine responses.

As a result, in cases like Rheumatoid Arthritis, it may assist decrease inflammation. Another function of the vagus nerve is to keep the neurological system in check. The vagus nerve sends messages to your brain when you're subjected to chilly temperatures while being outside. During this period, your body's natural response is to utilize breathing as a stress-reducing technique, moving you from sympathetic mode to parasympathetic mode. This activates the nerve with cryotherapy and helps you relax both physically and emotionally.

This technique was developed in Japan in the '70s and is still popular today. Because the vagus nerve reduces stress and improves mood, it may help relieve symptoms of depression. Nerve stimulation has short-term advantages including increased wakefulness, attention, memory recall, blood pressure reduction, and anxiety or tension reduction.

How would you feel if I told you that there is a way to completely change your perspective on taking care of your body, and it only requires three minutes out of your day? Whole-body cryotherapy (WBC) is a type of cold therapy performed by exposing the skin to temperatures ranging from -200°F to -250°F for three minutes.

Cryotherapy improves blood circulation immediately, allowing for proper oxygen and nutrient delivery to biological tissues while also enhancing the body's natural ability to eliminate impurities.

There are additional advantages to using cryotherapy if stimulating your vagus nerve isn't enough. Cryotherapy has a variety of benefits, including increasing your immune system function and helping athletes perform better. Athletes may enhance their performance when they include cryotherapy in their recovery program since it improves joint and muscle strength.

Because the muscles and tissues aren't totally frozen, you may begin exercising as soon as possible after treatment. Redistribution of blood occurs following vasodilation. Ice baths take longer to recover from than cryotherapy; this is due to the fact that muscles do not require time to heal themselves after freezing.

The body's metabolism is boosted by the low temperature in WBC, resulting in calories burned during the exercise. After a cryotherapy treatment, the body needs a lot of energy to warm up. During a two-to-three-minute session, 500-800 calories are burned for every person.

The body expends a significant amount of energy to return skin that has been cooled to around 35 degrees Fahrenheit to normal body temperature. Because the body's reactions are activated by perceived life-threatening situations, temperature control is not an issue since the body is compelled to utilize numerous powerful adaptive survival mechanisms that involve the body's most essential systems.

The blood vessels go back to their typical state after a session of cryotherapy, which then increases blood flow through the Capillaries and veins. This helps with collagen production as well as making your skin more elastic overtime by reducing cellulite or any fatty deposits on the surface.

Collagen is a protein that forms under the skin and gives your skin a youthful, smooth appearance. Collagen that has been activated reduces wrinkles and prevents new ones from forming.

Furthermore, because the tiny blood vessels are linked to facial blemishes, increasing blood flow might assist in the removal or healing of a variety of skin issues such as acne scars. Cryotherapy is a safe and natural method for relieving pain. Some people may experience a boost in mood for a few hours, whereas others may feel better for days. Regular cryotherapy treatments can help you keep your discomfort at bay.

To get the most out of cryotherapy, dress as little as possible to improve your skin's exposure to the cold. The teeth-chattering chill from head to toe stimulates the production of pain-relieving endorphins that heal tissues and cells.

People who feel down turn to cryotherapy because it releases endorphins and makes them happier. Endorphins interact with pain receptors and lessen the sensation of pain; cortisol levels drop, too, leading to an improved mood.

The vagus nerve has a powerful influence on your physical and mental health since it regulates both your breathing and heart rate as well as reducing inflammation throughout the body. Cryotherapy is an excellent method of delivering cryotherapy since it can be used for both acute and chronic injuries.

Cold thermogenesis is one of the biohacking techniques suggested by several authorities. Acute cold exposure activates both the vagus nerve and cholinergic and nitrergic neurons. When you're exposed to chilly temperatures, your sympathetic nervous system activity drops while your parasympathetic nervous system comes on. It restores and revitalizes you.

Cryotherapy is a quick and almost painless technique that can help with inflammation and pain reduction. It only takes 3 minutes, is dry, and does not require much preparation.

There have been reports of migraine relief with this approach. Furthermore, studies show that just three weeks of daily cryotherapy treatments can significantly reduce anxiety and depression symptoms. Ice-cold water, face immersion, deep breathing, and easy exercises may all help you get the most out of cryotherapy sessions by increasing vagal tone.

Ice baths

A temporary change in your body's fluid circulation (i.e., blood and lymph) occurs when you take an ice bath. The frigid water causes your blood vessels to constrict, but they will open up again once your body starts to warm back up post-bath.

The human body must excrete waste products through the skin, and this therapy aids in transporting them out of the system while also providing oxygen and nutrition to the muscles. Ice bath treatment is a coaching technique in which a large part of the human body, generally up to the chest, is immersed in an ice bath or iced water maintained at 50 to 59 degrees Fahrenheit for 10-15 minutes, usually following a high-intensity workout or competition.

Patients with multiple sclerosis or rheumatoid arthritis may find that supercooling the entire body for therapeutic reasons is beneficial. This method can help with a variety of illnesses. Ice baths boost your mood and attitude by stimulating your sympathetic and parasympathetic nervous systems, stress response, and recovery process.

When your body is exposed to the cold, sympathetic activity decreases while parasympathetic activity increases. It might be tough to teach your brain and body to accept cold treatment, but it's well worth the effort. Ice baths help with both physical recovery and mental, emotional, and psychological endurance. If you can get a hold of a cold tub and enjoy the feeling of immersion, dip in it once or twice a month.

Brown fat tissue is activated by low temperatures in your body. Brown fat helps to produce heat as your body consumes white fat. As a consequence, ice bathing on a regular basis can assist you keep weight off.

How to prepare an ice bath:

1. Purchase a few bags of ice at a supermarket or convenience shop.

2. Half-fill a bathtub or kiddie pool with cold water, being sure not to fill it too high. If you do, the ice will make the water level rise.

3. Fill the bathtub with ice, using half of what you think you'll need at first. The water should reach a temperature 55–60 °F (13–16 °C). To check the water's temperature, dip a thermometer into it.

4. Add extra ice if the water is too warm. Add some fresh water from the tap if the water is too cold.

5. Wearing swimming trunks will keep your delicate regions safe. Wear toe warmers or boots made of wetsuit fabric to keep your toes from getting cold.

6. Begin by submerging only the lower half of your body. Do not immerse more than the lower half of your body in ice baths when you initially begin.

7. To get used to the cold water, start by submerging only a few parts of your body. If that's too much, put ice in the bath after you've gotten in. You might find it easier to adjust this way.

8. Simply unwind in the tub. The point of an ice bath is not to cleanse your body, but rather to help you relax. You should also bring a sports drink with you in order replenish your electrolytes and hydration.

9. Distract yourself from the cold by reading a book or calling a friend.

10. Six to eight minutes is the perfect duration for your first cold water bath, and then you can work up to fifteen minutes over time. However, soaking in a cold bath for more than twenty minutes is detrimental to your health and muscles.

11. Fill it with cool water, followed by warm or hot water to rinse off the soap residue. After that, dry yourself with a clean towel so you can warm up. Use a clean towel to completely dry oneself after you've rinsed yourself. To keep warm while in the bath, cover yourself with a blanket or coat. Sip on some tea, coffee, or hot water with lemon while soaking in the tub.

Taking a cold bath may not sound like the most enjoyable experience, but it does have its benefits. By keeping three things in mind--breathing, focus and controlled exposure to cold--you can ease your body into the transition of colder weather slowly and effectively.

Did you know that submerging yourself can help to trigger a fundamental reflex known as the mammalian dive reflex? This is designed specifically to help you slow down and conserve energy. Not to mention, it is easy to do and can have a big impact on your vagus if done regularly!

The ice bath also aids in the reduction of heating and humidity. Although this has nothing to do with the vagus nerve, it is an intriguing fact. Taking an ice bath before a race in which the temperature or humidity are expected to rise is usually beneficial. It improves performance by lowering the temperature of the lower core body by a few degrees.

Ice baths have their own set of challenges and precautions to follow. Hypothermia is a potential danger that comes with any exposure to extreme cold, and ice baths are no exception. An ice bath can cause the body temperature to go down, which can limit blood circulation by restricting blood vessels and increasing pressure in the veins.

The first symptoms of hypothermia occur when people are immersed in 41°F water for 10 to 20 minutes. Cold does not relax muscles; instead, it causes them to contract. When used on tense or tight muscles, particularly the lower back or neck, cold can exacerbate pain by causing them to contract.

Consult with your doctor if you have high blood pressure or cardiovascular illness before trying any of the following alternatives to ice baths, which are known to speed up recovery: massages, gentle stretching, foam rolling, or dynamic range of motion exercises like yoga.

Since cold weather constricts blood vessels and reduces blood flow to the arms and legs, the heart must work harder to pump blood through constricted capillaries. This can exacerbate heart problems in patients who have a history of high blood pressure or heart disease.

When the water temperature is below 59 degrees, immersing yourself in an ice bath too rapidly or for a long duration can shock your body and cause blood pressure and heart rate to rise, making it unpleasant.

If you're considering vagus nerve stimulation, always talk to your doctor first. They can help make sure ice baths are right for you and give guidance on how often to partake in them. That said, when done correctly, taking an icy plunge can do wonders for stimulating the vagus nerve—benefits include a calmer mind and lessened stress levels.

Deep Breathing

Another approach to activate your vagus nerve is to breathe deeply and slowly. It has been discovered that by stimulating the vagus nerve, anxiety may be relieved and the parasympathetic system may function more effectively.

Each minute, the average person takes 10 to 14 breaths. To relieve tension, take approximately six breaths every minute, according on my recommendation of deep breathing from the diaphragm and extended and slow exhalations and inhalations. When you do this, your stomach should extend outward. This is essential for stimulating the vagus nerve and relaxing.

When you concentrate on your breath instead of the pain, stressor, or anxiety, it allows your brain to take a break from processing those thoughts. The human brain can only process one thought at a time, and by focusing on something else - like your breathing - you are effectively giving it a break. Breath-holding often leads to an increased sense of fear or anxiety due to triggering the fight-flight-freeze reaction in our bodies.

To learn how to do deep breathing, breathe in and out through your nose. Remember to take a slow breath and try for six breaths per minute. Deepen your breathing by filling your belly button with air as you inhale. Imagine expanding your tummy and rib cage while exhaling.

If you want to feel relaxed and invigorated, exhale for longer than you inhale. For every two counts you breathe in, breath out for four. At the top of your inhale, pause for one count and do likewise at the bottom of your exhale. The relaxation reaction is more likely to occur when triggering it with deep breaths. So sit or lie down comfortably and take as many deep breaths as possible before holding it in for a second or two then letting go; repeat this five to ten times more.

As you inhale, expand your abdomen fully. Remember to lengthen both your exhales and inhales gradually. To increase the relaxation response, it is necessary to slow down your exhalation as you progress in breath control exercises.

Lowering the sympathetic nervous system and strengthening the parasympathetic nervous system may help to alleviate anxiety, as some experts suggest. One way to do this is through slow, deep breathing exercises from your belly button, which Yoruba practitioners recommend. When inhaling, allow your stomach area to expand outward like a balloon filling with air. As you exhale slowly, let your stomach fall inward towards your spine.

Gargling

By gargling with water as hard as you can first thing in the morning, you are stimulating the vagus nerve. The muscles located at the back of your throat are controlled by this particular nerve. To determine if you're doing it correctly, look for tearing eyes. You should aim to do this multiple times throughout the day.

To help improve the vagal nerve pathways, drink large glasses of water each day and gargle after each sip until the glass is empty. Gargling theory activates the vagus nerve and stimulates the gastrointestinal system by contracting those muscles at the back of your throat.

Meditation

It has been shown in some studies that meditation can actually help to indirectly stimulate the vagus nerve, making it an excellent way to reduce tension and increase mindfulness-awareness over time. In particular, love-kindness and mindfulness meditation have been found to be particularly effective at enhancing heart rate variability, which is connected to vagal tone.

If you want to improve your health, some researchers recommend a minimum of twenty minutes of meditation each day. They believe that the calming effect is caused by deep breathing, which directly stimulates the vagus nerve and associated rest-and-digest neural activity. Find a way to meditate that you genuinely enjoy so that it doesn't feel like a chore.

If you want to meditate, find a way that works for you whether it be through videos or an app. Then, decide when the best time of day would be to work this into your schedule, and stick with it. If having someone else there makes it more likely that you'll do it daily, ask a friend to join you or look into groups.

Meditation, particularly loving-kindness meditation, can lead to increased positive emotions towards yourself and others. These improved positive emotions result in increased social proximity as well as an increase in vagal tone. Meditation has been found to boost the parasympathetic nervous system by lowering the heart rate and breathing, loosening the muscles of the abdomen, and slowing brain function - whether it's a guided meditation session or a regular habit of sitting and watching your breath.

The vagus nerve is responsible for communicating to the brain whether or not the body is safe. By focusing on positive, loving thoughts, we can help stimulate the vagus nerve and send messages to the brain that it is safe to relax.

Yoga

Yoga has been shown in studies to improve digestion and reduce anxiety by increasing the levels of GABA. The vagal tone may be increased by raising GABA levels. Regular moderate exercise, such as yoga, has been found to increase gastric motility, or stomach muscle contractions that aid in the passage of food through the digestive tract.

The regular practice of yoga has many benefits for both the mind and body. In addition to promoting a good mood and reducing anxiety, it also activates the Vagus Nerve and the parasympathetic nervous system.

Baroreceptors, which are pressure sensors in the heart and neck that send messages to the brain to activate the Vagus Nerve through slow, deep breathing, are activated by yoga.

Slow, rhythmic breathing with roughly equal inhale and exhale durations while practicing yoga can enhance the effect considerably. Yoga is similar to meditation, so whether you participate in a class, use a mobile app, or watch online videos on your own, it doesn't matter since it's part of your daily routine.

Tai Chi

Tai chi is a graceful form of exercise that was developed in China and is still practiced today. It comprises of a series of slow, deliberate motions that are followed by deep breathing. Tai chi, often known as tai chi chuan, is a non-competitive type of stretching and fitness.

Tai chi is a martial arts style that teaches you to move through space. It starts with your posture, which should be as upright as possible while still being comfortable. The next set of movements builds on the previous ones, so you'll never stop moving. Tai Chi is not Yoga. Yoga has various physical postures, breathing techniques, and meditation exercises. Tai chi has been found to increase vagus nerve activity while lowering heart rates, blood pressure, blood glucose levels, and cholesterol levels.

Singing and Chanting

The vagus nerve has been shown to respond positively to singing and chanting, which in turn calms the body. If you feel shy about singing in public, try doing it in the shower or while driving with the music on low volume. You can use any type of music or chant that you enjoy.

The goal is to create a sense of peace while also emitting purifying, beneficial vibrations. Working the muscles in the back of the throat activates the vagus nerve. The vagus nerve links your voice chords and muscles at the rear of your throat.

Singing, humming, and/or chanting can all be used to activate and stimulate these muscles. According to research, reciting fundamental mantras has a significant impact on the vagus nerve, which explains why it has a tranquilizing effect on the entire being. Singing in tune might have a greater impact. If this isn't your thing, you may use "OM" chanting in yoga or mediation as an add-on. Make sure you sing loudly and have fun!

Physical Activity

Exercise not only strengthens your brain by aiding in the production of growth hormone, but also Burlington's mitochondria. In addition, it can help give you clarity and better cognitive function as well as improve mental health by stimulating the vagus nerve.

Exercise is crucial for brain health, and there are many different types of exercises that can help. Some of the most common forms of exercise include walking, weightlifting, and sprinting. However, it's important to find an activity or workout routine that you enjoy so that you're more likely to stick with it on a regular basis. Exercise can not only improve your vagal tone but also boost your overall happiness levels.

Examples of exercise regimes can be:

· Heavy weightlifting one to four times per week

· Take your dog for a walk or play tug-of-war with him. Engage in mild activity to keep the metabolism going and aid weight loss. Make time for some (HIIT) high-intensity interval training (HIRT) sessions once or twice per week. You may do this exercise either in a group or alone using online videos as guidance. It promotes not just improved vagus nerve activity during exercise, but also after workout recovery.

· Taking speedy walks or lightly jogging for half an hour each day is a great way to stay healthy. Choose the time of day that works best for you, and pick locations that you like going to, whether they are by the water or in nature. If having someone reliable beside you helps make sure you stick with this beneficial habit, ask a friend to join you.

Massages

Massaging several distinct parts of the body might stimulate the vagus nerve. Foot massages, often known as reflexology, have been found to enhance vagal tone and heart rate variability while reducing the sympathetic "fight or flight" response.

To keep seizures at bay, doctors can massage the carotid sinus—a cluster of nerves surrounding the carotid artery on either side of your throat. The recipient lies down with their chin raised and allowed the doctor to apply pressure to areas near the jaw. Carrying out this method should be done with monitoring equipment in place.

Massage improves vagal tone and stimulates the lymphatic system. It also helps your entire body's blood flow, including the billions of sensitive nerve endings in your hands and feet, which is why it's so beneficial for just 10 minutes each day.

To improve your vagal tone and increase vagal activity, massage yourself regularly or get a professional massage. This nerve can also be stimulated by pressuremassage, which can aid weight gain in newborns by stimulating the gut (which is largely mediated by vagus nerve stimulation).

Massage guns

A portable massage gun is a gadget that you can charge and use to thump away at your muscles for as long as you'd like, sometimes up to 2500 times per minute. We're not entirely sure how these technologies affect the human body just yet, but they may help relax painful muscles by activating the GTO (Golgi tendon organ). The GTO is a muscular component that helps prevent muscle contraction and tension changes.

The massage gun is located at the myotendinous junction, which connects a muscle to its tendon. It is effectively like having a masseuse available to you whenever you want or need one. You are essentially changing your brain's ability to detect stiffness or looseness in soft tissue, such as muscles, tendons, and fascia.

Massage guns have come a long way since they were first created-- all the way from just vibrating the muscle to help it relax, to slightly kneading it. When you use a massage gun, either your therapist's hands or the device itself will let you know which muscles are tensed up so that your brain can learn to release that tension.

A massage gun is a tool used to massage muscles and increase blood flow, which carries nutrients to the muscles while removing blood that has built up in them—a typical occurrence that can lead to edema in the limbs after long periods of inactivity. If you apply the gun just after a workout, it might assist remove metabolites and waste products from your body.

Remember that, while the cold may help aching shoulders recover more quickly, excessive stimulation might be harmful. It's best to keep it in a modest area because it's a powerful instrument. People think they must remain on it if they find an area that hurts. They could be passing over a bony prominence or a vein-artery nerve bundle, for example. Neuropathy and numbness in the hands can result from cutting these sensitive regions over time.

A massage gun is no match for a skilled massage practitioner. It has no way of telling the difference between bone, muscle, fascia, and nerve; it doesn't know if you're injured; and it can't tell whether tissue is too tight or too loose. As a result, you should talk to a medical professional before purchasing one. You may be shown how to use it at home as desired. Some models come with different heads that you should use on different regions of your body, so keep that in mind as well.

Acupuncture

Acupuncture, when applied to areas in the head, ears, and neck, has a comparable relaxing effect to massaging pressure points. If you want to see an acupuncturist, work with a reputable acupuncture specialist who is licensed by your state.

Theinsertion of clean needles is a critical part of acupuncture to prevent issues such as infection.BY stimulating the Vagus Nerve, practiced correctly, ear acupuncture has shown in Traditional Chinese Medicine be an effective method for several thousand years. As opposed to more common methods which utilize needles, pseudo-acupunctureInstead uses toothpicks.

If seeing a professional acupuncturist is not an option, the layman may do this at home. The vagus nerve innervates your tragus, auricle, and skin surrounding your inner ear canal. You can elicit a response by tapping a toothpick over these locations on your face.

Chiropractic treatment

Your neurological system is flexible. Try bending a plastic fork gently without breaking it. It will return to its original shape. The more you repeat this, the more plastic will bend. It's the same with your neurological system. As your brain becomes accustomed to its defensive state, survival becomes your default option.

Many health problems such as high blood pressure, indigestion, autoimmune flare-ups, chronic ear infections, insomnia and more are caused by living in survival mode. It's hard to develop and repair when you're only trying to survive.

Regular chiropractic treatments cause the activity of your vagus nerve to rise. HRV has been shown in studies to improve in patients who received regular chiropractic treatment. HRV may be used to measure your neurological system, which is responsible for controlling and coordinating your heart.

Your body is a self-regulating and self-healing system. Your nervous system controls and organizes your own healing and self-regulation skills. Your capacity to cope with life's challenges determines your chances of survival and recovery. HRV is an excellent method for detecting nervous system adaptability.

If you can keep a balance between the PNS and SNS parts of your nervous system, you will be able to heal and recover more easily. Because the vagus nerve is connected to vital nerves in the spine and upper neck, chiropractors place a lot of emphasis on it.

The health of the vagus nerve is shaped by the state of one's spine. If there is a problem with the spine, messages sent from and toward the vagus nerve are disrupted. Chiropractors pay attention to spinal alignment and mobility in order to promote better vagus nerve functioning.

Chiropractic adjustments that directly impact the function of the vagal nerve have a significant role to play in reducing chronic illness. The spinal column houses all nerves, so even a slight misalignment can cause big problems for the neurological system. Keep it functioning properly with regular chiropractic adjustments!

The eighth nerve has a unique function; it connects to numerous organs, glands, and tissues as it courses from the brain to the cervical spine. It's important to note where this nerve leaves the neck. This nerve is affected by both positive and negative influences of C1 vertebrae, therefore a customized chiropractic treatment is required.

The better the Vagus nerve may be influenced non-invasively, the better. Always consult your doctor before receiving alternative therapy and make sure you do so from an expert.

Osteopathy treatment

Osteopathic manipulation helps to restore the normal functioning of the vagus nerve and assist digestion by releasing soft tissue and joint restrictions in the cranium's base and top neck. Through muscles in the middle ear, the vagus nerve and facial nerve regulate strain on the ossicle bones caused by tension on muscles in the face.

Osteopathy is a therapy that treats people by manipulating their bodies and tissues. Touching others can be beneficial on both the physical and mental levels, as it causes the release of oxytocin in the brain. Oxytocin is sometimes referred to as the "cuddle hormone" because it produces feelings of warmth, affection, and security.

Oxytocin has anti-stress effects, including lowering cortisol levels and assisting sleep. It lowers anxiety and promotes tissue development and regeneration. The primary benefit of the Osteopathic touch is to assist the body in regaining its homeostatic equilibrium, allowing it to heal more effectively.

Osteopathic practitioners focus on areas of dysfunction and pain. The ability to palpate--or detect by touch--is something that osteopathic practitioners learn. The cranial rhythm is created when cerebrospinal fluid enters and leaves the central nervous system. If you can't perceive the cranial beat, consult an osteopathic practitioner; they'll help your body heal naturally.

The greatest benefit of osteopathic palpation is that practitioners frequently feel the same things you do in your body, without you having to tell them. If you have joint discomfort, for example, an osteopath can check for joint stiffness, so even if you forgot to mention it to your practitioner, they may still discover it on their own.

Chiropractic treatment VS Osteopathic treatment

You may be asking yourself what the distinction is between chiropractic and osteopathic treatment, as well as how it affects the vagus nerve differently, after hearing everything Haven just said.

Osteopathy is a form of alternative medicine that focuses on myofascial release, manual adjustments, and other physical manipulation of the bones and muscles. nThe numerous advantages of working with an osteopath are debatable, although they may vary depending on your health issue.

As a result, it is critical that you feel at ease with and trust your osteopath. Osteopaths specialize in musculoskeletal problems, so if you have arthritis, postural imbalances, joint/muscle strains, or other diseases such as sciatica or whiplash, they can assist. Some osteopaths believe that the spine has an impact on the rest of the body, particularly the immune system.

Chiropractic caretakers focus on keeping the body healthy instead of merely diagnosing and treating illnesses. This means you may receive more effective treatment for immune system or hormone-related problems.

Because these side effects lessen the nervous system's ability to function properly, chiropractic care focuses on the joints and spine as well as the entire nervous system. By using spinal adjustments, chiropractors can help restore joint function while supporting the nervous system. Medicine and surgery are not needed for this type of treatment plan.

A chiropractor is a doctor who focuses on the health and well-being of the spine. They specialize in conservative treatment for a variety of spinal problems and illnesses. By applying a safe, regulated, and targeted force to the joints or muscles, a chiropractic adjustment restores normal mobility and function.

Chiropractors can help with a wide range of ailments, despite the fact that the vast majority of people think they only treat neck and back pain. Chiropractors may help with headaches and migraines, recurrent injuries, lower back discomfort, sciatica problems, arthritis pains, and sports injuries.

The primary distinction between chiropractors and osteopaths is that whereas chiropractors are primarily focused on the joints and spine, osteopaths are concerned with the entire body and how it works. Osteopaths practice holistic medicine, which means they consider all contributing factors to your pain or pinched nerve symptoms.

When you visit a chiropractor or an osteopath, they will ask you about your discomfort, when it started, what you were doing before the pain began, and other things. They'll also inspect you and make a diagnosis based on your symptoms. You may be given several treatments depending on your issues.

To summarize, chiropractors use manipulative therapies to realign your spine and joint positions in order to improve nerve function and relieve pain. In contrast, osteopaths utilize massages, manipulation, and stretching to restore the body's structure in order to enhance nerve activity and blood flow.

What is the best way to induce a vagal tone? Both of these approaches stimulate the vagus nerve. It all depends on your concerns and your weakest spots. It's wise to choose the proper therapy by consulting with your doctor about it.

Cupping

Cupping has become increasingly popular as a form of alternative medicine after Michael Phelps was photographed with well-circumscribed bruises at one of his competitions. Cupping is one of the aspects of traditional Chinese medicine (TCM). The imbalance and disregulation of the vagus nerve might be relieved by this technique.

The ability of cupping to improve circulation by drawing blood and lymph away from the skin is due to suction. Cupping can help with a variety of issues, including aches and pains, colds and flues, as well as airborne allergies. Cupping may aid in the reduction of headaches, migraines, anxiety, and cellulite breakage and removal.

The improvement of blood circulation from this therapy helps to ease muscular tension and allow for better overall blood flow and cell healing. It also assists in the formation of new connective tissues and blood vessels in the tissue. Even though it boasts many advantages, you must have an Oriental medicine practitioner do a comprehensive body examination before deciding on this therapy as your treatment option.

Not all problems are caused by a single source of stasis, and we must address everyone's requirements individually. Cupping leaves bruise-like marks that should disappear after ten to fourteen days, depending on your immune system.

For the first 48 hours, treat yourself as if you were sick by restricting your activity, eating solid food, drinking alcohol, or using drugs since your tolerance may be low and result in serious issues as your system tries to detox. Please wait at least twenty-four hours after therapy before taking a shower or exposing your skin to extreme temperatures, hot or cold.

The two types of cupping are dry and wet. Dry cupping uses suction only, while wet cupping may also include therapeutic bleeding that is controlled. The approach used will be decided based on your practitioner's professional opinion, your medical condition, and what you as the patient prefer.

Suction may be used only or, in some cases, through the use of fire. The cups begin to suction against the skin once the fire is inserted into the cup and has consumed all of the oxygen inside.

A cup is placed on the skin and then heated or suctioned during cupping therapy. Alcohol, plants, or paper is frequently inserted straight into the cup to allow for a fire to start. The fire source is switched off, and the heated cup is applied to your skin with the open side facing toward you.

When you place the heated cup on your skin, the air within cools, creating a vacuum that draws the skin and muscle upward into the cup. Your skin may become red as blood vessels adjust to the change in pressure. For dry cupping, you leave the cup in place for a specific length of time, usually between five and ten minutes.

Cups are usually only left in place for a few minutes with wet cupping before the practitioner removes them. They then make a tiny incision to draw blood. Following the removal of the cups, the practitioner may apply ointment and bandages to the previously cupped regions. This helps prevent infection. Acupuncture treatments are sometimes combined with cupping.

To yield the best benefits, it is encouraged that you fast or eat light meals for two to three hours before your cupping session. Because the cups may be used to apply pressure to important acupressure points, the technique may help with digestive issues, skin conditions, and other ailments that respond well to acupressure.

After undergoing cupping therapy, you may experience redness and circles around the rim of the cup. You may feel discomfort near the incision sites or dizzy and confused shortly after your treatment. While infection is rare, it is still a possibility, as well as scarring and bruising.

This is an established phenomena that will go away on its own. A practitioner should wear an apron, disposable gloves, and goggles, or glasses that provide adequate eye protection. To defend themselves from diseases like hepatitis, they should also get vaccines on a regular basis. Always do your homework regarding practitioners to assure your safety.

If you're having any of these issues, see your therapist. Pregnant women, children, the elderly with delicate skin, and menstruating ladies are prohibited from cupping. If you're taking blood thinners, avoid cupping. You should avoid cupping if you have a sunburn, skin irritation or ulceration, internal organ disease or recent trauma. And as previously stated, be sure to inform your doctor about your treatment plan.

Moxibustion

The discovery that temperature has a profound effect on the human body has given rise to moxibustion, more commonly known as "moxa." Acupuncture and moxibustion have been used together for centuries in order to stimulate blood flow, get rid of sickness, and improve overall health; however, they are not nearly as popular in western cultures.

Moxa is an Ancient Chinese Healing technique that involves the use of dried mugwort plant to stimulate acupuncture sites and energy channels by creating penetrating heat.

Moxibustion, which involves the application of moxa to the skin directly or over a medium such as ginger or salt, on acupuncture needles, or in the form of cigar-shaped sticks allowing practitioners to stroll around the body and administer moxa as desired during treatment, is one type of TCM therapy.

This supplement is wonderful for boosting your system, and it's frequently used in clinical therapies. Many people suffer from low energy levels or what is known as chronic cold conditions, so this supplement can be a great help.

Tui na Massage

Tui na is a Chinese manipulative therapy that uses hands-on techniques to restore balance within the body. This type of treatment is often used for musculoskeletal issues, but it can also be helpful for physiological conditions that are linked to digestion and menstruation.

Tui Na is a form of massage that can be either gentle or strong, making it perfect for anyone. This massage strives to be both relaxing and invigorating by using motions such as gliding, kneading, rocking, pressing, rubbing, and rolling. Tui Na goes beyond Western massages by working on the body's energy level rather than just the muscles, bones, and joints.

Tui Na massage combines the hands of a Tui Na practitioner with the energy of the person he or she is treating. During their therapeutic session, experts in this style use their hands to feel the client's energy and then alter it and distribute it throughout the body. Acupuncture, Chinese herbal medicines, moxibustion, and cupping are all common Tui Na massage treatments. Tui Na massage is beneficial for individuals who suffer from persistent neck discomfort.

Aromatherapy

Essential oils are extracted from plants. The plants are crushed or steamed to extract the oils, and fragrant oils of various qualities are created as a result. Plant parts such as fruit, leaves, flowers, and bark are used to make essential oils.

Aromatherapy using essential oils to produce a desired fragrance has been used since ancient times and for good reason- it works! The vagus nerve is one of the ways that essential oils can be useful in treating various illnesses. This method usually increasesvagal tone, leaving a calming effect that aids in sleep and digestion.

scent plays a role in our five senses, and it can have a strong impact on how we think and feel. Aromatherapy has been shown to help relax the vagus nerve, which is responsible for regulating the body's fight-or-flight response. This can lead to feelings of relaxation and improved digestion.

The intensity and pleasantness of the scent may be changed to affect a variety of functions in the body. This is why aromatherapy can help to relax the vagus nerve. When receptors in the nose are stimulated, sensory impulses are transmitted to the brain. The vagus nerve transmits information to the limbic system in your brain, which helps you relax and manages behavioral and emotional reactions.

The limbic system can be calmed through the vagus nerve, leading to more manageable emotional and behavioral responses. Some of the oils used are lemongrass, peppermint, lavender, and eucalyptus. They can be either rubbed on directly or burned using a diffuser or burner.

If you chose to apply them directly to the skin, try the following technique:

1. Take a seat or lie down.

2. Place a few drops of your desired essential oil onto your fingers, then massage it into the left side of your neck starting from your clavicle and working up. Repeat this process until you've covered the entire neck area. To intensify the effects of the oil, warm up the bottle in your hands for a few minutes before using.

3. Carry on with step 2 while taking slow, deep breaths.

Essential oils can assist to stimulate the vagus nerve, which may enhance your mood. The fragrant air is also therapeutic.

Socializing

Focusing on good social connections, according to a study, improves positive feelings and increases vagal tone. Laughter has been shown to improve mood and heart health. Furthermore, vagus nerve stimulation frequently causes people to laugh as a side effect, suggesting that the two are related and have an impact on one another.

Laughter improves your mood and overall outlook, strengthens your immune system against sickness, and even has the power to help facilitate emotional healing. When you laugh, your brain releases endorphins which are designed to produce positive feelings in order relieve stress. In other words: laughter makes you feel good!

There is research to suggest that the vagal circuit and emotional regulation are linked. This means that improving your emotional regulation can lead to a boost in happiness and overall well-being. So, no matter what is going on in the world around you, make sure you take time to interact with others, laugh, and enjoy life.

Laughter has been shown to improve heart health by increasing levels of beta-endorphins and nitric oxide, both of which are known to be beneficial to the circulatory system. The cardiac vagal tone may be enhanced by diaphragmatic movements produced by laughter, according on studies.

Laughter not only helps to minimize SNS activity by relieving emotional stress, but it also aids in the release of hostile, undesirable energy that has built up as tension in the body owing to prior SNS overstimulation.

Sleeping on your right side

Reducing Vagus Nerve activation occurs when a person sleeps on their back, but more stimulation of the vagus nerve is had by sleeping on one's right side as opposed to the left. The sympathetic nervous system controls the fight-or-flight response. As part of this reaction, both heart rate and blood pressure rise.

Most cardiac patients experience worsened heart failure, chest discomfort, and arrhythmias when the sympathetic nervous system is activated. When it comes to sleeping and sympathetic stimulation, research indicates that sleeping on the right side is more beneficial. Nobody wants to feel like their heart isn't pounding properly.

Sleeping on your right side increases the amount of blood ejected by your heart. Gravity may help to maximize cardiac function by moving the heart into the chest's central area. This might be due to increased venous return and decreased cardiac and respiratory pressures, both of which are favorable for cardiac output.

Prayer

I'm not sure if this is for everyone, but it can assist stimulate the vagus nerve, especially the rosary prayer, if you are religious. It appears to improve cardiac rhythms by lowering diastolic blood pressure and improving HRV.

Because one rosary bead takes roughly 10 seconds to read, readers are compelled to breathe at 10-second intervals, including both in and out breaths, increasing HRV and subsequently vagus activity. Faith is a wonderful antidote to stress; it's well known that reducing stress raises vagal activation, which aids immunity.

So, if faith works for you, add it to your list of stress-reducing strategies. Someone who understands and embraces prayer as a powerful force can stimulate the vagus nerve significantly. Someone new to prayer, on the other hand, may not get a strong vagal reaction. So, certainly, if you believe in its power, prayer can activate the vagus nerve.

Coffee enemas

A cup of coffee in the morning is a must-have for many who rely on caffeine to get through the day. Many people, on the other hand, learn that their morning cup of coffee improves their bowel movements. This is why some individuals employ coffee enemas as a treatment.

We recommend that patients with brain degeneration perform daily coffee enemas. This helps to stimulate the vagus nerve, which is responsible for intestinal motility. Caffeine acts on cholinergic receptors in the gut, promoting bowel movements and overall general health.

Many patients notice that their bowel function improves over time, and they can eventually stop using enemas. Taking enemas rather than attempting to have a bowel movement on your own, on the other hand, might damage your intestines and make it more difficult to avoid using them in the future. As a result, reducing enema usage over time is crucial.

The enemas help encourage positive changes in the pathways of the vagal system. When you drink coffee, it leads to your gallbladder contracting and allows waste products from liver metabolism to be released into your colon so that they can eventually be eliminated. Unfortunately, there are also always harmful chemicals and pollutants present in our food, air, and water supply.

Coffee enemas can be used by anybody to assist with the stimulation of the liver and the purification of waste materials and impurities from their bodies. Coffee enemas can be used instead of stimulant laxatives to cleanse the intestine before an endoscopy. According to study, coffee enemas are a feasible way to prepare the intestines without causing significant side effects.

Although more research is necessary, coffee enemas are becoming increasingly popular for bowel preparation. Cramps, pressure, and fullness are common side effects of a coffee enema. As caffeine is a main ingredient in coffee, you may also feel unsteady or have cardiac palpitations. To avoid dehydration after your procedure, drink lots of water.

Follow these steps to prepare a coffee enema at home:

I. To make one liter of coffee, add 2 teaspoons of ground coffee to a standard coffee machine. This should yield around 4 cups of 8-ounce coffee. Make sure that the finished product is free from any grounds.

II. Allow enough time for the coffee to cool down to room temperature. For the enema, never use hot or even warm water.

III. Organization is key when preparing to infuse water into your body. Place towels on a bed, couch or any other soft location where you will be comfortable lying down on your left side. being close to a restroom is essential in case you need to relieve yourself immediately after the procedure since digestive systems are known to react differently when fluids enter the ileum (final section of the small intestine).

IV. Most drugstores will have an enema device available for purchase. These usually come with a water bottle and tubing that can be inserted into the rectum. To use, insert the coffee mixture into the rectum using the device.

V. To ensure ease of insertion, a water-based lubricant can be applied to the tube.

VI. Fill the rectum with as much of the one-liter coffee or water cocktail as possible. It's not ideal to try to force everything in.

VII. For ten to fifteen minutes, the solution should be retained in the rectum. When enemas are retained for this long, they are most effective. After, a person should try to use the restroom.

VIII. A second enema may be required if the initial one does not have a significant impact. It's important not to repeat an enema therapy too often since doing so can cause the loss of electrolytes, which are essential for keeping fluid balance in the body.

Long-term diarrhea caused by frequent enemas can create unsafe electrolyte imbalances; therefore, anyoen experiencing this should consult a medical professional.

Because non-organic coffee can contain hazardous pesticides, prepare your enema using organic coffee. The stronger the coffee, the more it stimulates the vagus nerve. Water that has been filtered or distilled is ideal. Coffee should be boiled for around ten minutes before straining out the grounds.

Before using, allow the coffee to cool down to room temperature. To check if the coffee is cooled sufficiently, immerse your entire hand in it for five seconds. Some people instead choose phosphate enemas for their first time. Enemas are best done with medical supervision as there is a risk of low electrolyte levels in the body that can cause harm.

Because you are administering an enema in your own home, bacterial infection is a possibility. For this procedure, expert medical care and cleanliness are required. To stimulate the vagus nerve for as long as possible, the enema should be tough to hold. If you're sensitive to coffee, use a weaker brew for longer retention. As you get more experience with enemas, increase the strength of the coffee used.

Although coffee enemas can have several benefits, they also come with a range of risks that are important to be aware of before trying them. If you are caffeine-sensitive or using medications that could interact with caffeine, coffee enemas might not be suitable for you. Possible side effects of colon cleansing include rectal burns, nausea, vomiting, cramps, bloating and dehydration – as well as more serious issues such as intestinal perforation or infection from incorrectly cleaned equipment.

However, coffee enemas may worsen certain illnesses such as abdominal hernia, blood vessel illness, congestive heart failure, Crohn's disease, and diverticulitis. If you have any of the following chronic conditions or gastrointestinal issues – intestinal tumors, severe anemia hemorrhoids,, or ulcerative colitis – it is best to avoid coffee enemas altogether. Consult with your doctor to make the decision that is right for you.

Coffee enemas, in addition to a plant-based diet high in potassium and low in salt, are used by the Gerson therapy. To cure and detoxify the body, he recommended coffee enemas in conjunction with a diet high in potassium and low in salt.

Gerson believed that coffee enemas were a way to detox the body from any poison living inside it. According to Gerson, coffee enemas not only boost cell production but also promote better tissue health and circulation. He further claimed that it strengthens immunity and helps with cell growth.

Binaural beats

When you hear two tones, one in each ear, that differ slightly in frequency, your brain creates a rhythm based on the difference. This is known as a binaural beat. The tones must be listened to one at a time, one in each ear. Binaural beats have been investigated in music and are sometimes used to tune pianos and organs.

Binaural rhythms have shown to produce the same mentally calming state as meditation, but much quicker. They are also said to help with pain management by reducing anxiety, tension and promoting relaxation and creativity--all while fostering happy moods.

When you listen to a sound with a specific frequency, your brain waves can synchronize with it. According to the theory, binaural beats may help create the frequency required for your brain to produce similar waves as those experienced during meditation. I just learnt that a gadget has been developed to achieve this.

The Nervana device improves calm and reduces tension by claims to stimulate the vagus nerve while a person listens to music. The stimulation reportedly causes neurotransmitters, including serotonin and oxytocin, to be released in the brain.

Nervana is a black box that you plug your music device into. It then sends the signal of the music being played to both earphones, but delivers the regular music to one and an altered signal to the other, syncing according to the rhythm.

To avoid any ambiguity, the earphones are color-coded; blue for the left ear providing electrical stimulation. The Nervana'sFlorida-based creators recommend using it twice daily for 15 to 45 minutes each time.

Chewing Gum

The act of chewing gum increases the release of a hormone called Cholecystokinin (CCK) from your gut. This, in turn, helps the Vagus Nerve communicate with your brain. The vagus nerve impulses back and forth between your brain are required for CCK to reduce food intake and appetite overall. Gum chewing may assist enhance CCK release; however, most gum is unhealthy and contains added sugars and other additives, so choose the healthier alternatives.

Expose yourself to sunlight!

UVA radiation activates the Vagus Nerve via an increase in melanocyte-stimulating hormone (MSH) production. UVB rays stimulate the number of MSH receptors present throughout the body, allowing for increased MSH production. Sun exposure may be very damaging if not properly limited, therefore applying a good sunscreen is always advised.

Sun protection does not mean these beneficial rays are blocked completely but rather are absorber gradually, lessening the harm done to the skin.

At-home methods of natural stimulation can increase vagal tone. You don't always need to see a professional in order to do some self-care practices that improve your vagus nerve function. Improving your vagal tone can lead to better moods, digestion, and physical health overall.

Daily Vagus exercises

The following are some of the exercises that may be done to stimulate the vagus nerve. Some of them use the vagus nerve, while others are created specifically to cure certain illnesses.

The Valsalva Maneuver

For an immediate vagal nerve stimulation, do the Valsala maneuver. Be warned that you may feel dizzy, so it's best to sit down first. Inhale deeply then close your mouth and nose so no air can escape. Try to exhale without opening your lips or nose."

To find out whether the air is flowing properly, check to see if there is any resistance. Continue for 15-20 seconds before letting off the air and taking a normal breath. Repeat five times in total. The increased pressure within your chest cavity causes your vagal tone to rise. It's possible that sitting or squatting would help you open up more.

The Valsalva technique is a simple but effective way to combat supraventricular tachycardia, or problems with the electrical signals in your heart. The exercise is named after 17th-century physician Antonio Maria Valesio, who described it as a treatment for regulatingsb blood pressure and heart rate. Here's how it works: when you blow into closed lips, the pressure in your chest and belly rises.

Your blood pressure rises for a short while when you do this Arm and Shoulder Stretch because your heart pumps less blood with each beat. But don't worry, your blood pressure gradually normalizes as you go along. You may even find that your heart rate increases towards the end of the exercise!

As your heart beats faster and blood rushes back to it, you may notice your blood pressure increase. This is normal and should gradually return to normal. However, if you have a cardiac illness, only use the Valsalva technique if directed by your doctor. Although it is uncommon, the procedure has the potential to induce chest discomfort and other cardiac rhythm issues. This maneuver can sometimes induce a surge in pressure behind the eyes.If you have retinopathy, which is damage to the retina of the eye, or an implanted lens, do not attempt this.

Exercises for Postural defects

The following exercises improve your thoracic spine flexibility, making it easier to move the joints between the ribs and sternum. You'll be able to take deeper breaths, correct forward head posture, and reduce scoliosis.

By improving your breathing pattern with these exercises, you tell the brain that you are safe and that your visceral organs are functioning properly, allowing ventral vagal activation to be easier. In addition, a forward head posture reduces the amount of breathing space in the upper chest.

Knees out and away from the body in a dogmatic posture is present when you are attempting to assert yourself. Knees together and close to your chest, as well as overly erect shoulders, indicate that you're forcing yourself into an alpha position unnecessarily (even if it's effective). Knees out and away from the body are signs of kyphosis or forward head posture (FHP), which is a condition in which the trapezius and sternocleidomastoid muscles are malfunctioning and lead to significant health issues. Bad posture has various effects, one of which is a forward head position. People lose their ideal stance with age, and they may experience breathing difficulties on a regular basis.

The difficulties that come with FHP are often not medicalized because doctors naturalize them as an entirely age-related process. Though impossible to cure, there are ways to ease the pain of living with this condition. When you have FHP, your neck will gravity-sink which in turn pushes your head forward from its original position. The distance between your heart and lungs shortens when upper chest compression occurs

Forward head posture also hampers the functioning of muscles that aid in the lift of the first rib during inhalation, making breathing more difficult. As FHP gets worse, you lose a greater amount of your respiratory capacity. People who suffer from respiratory difficulties such as asthma and chronic obstructive pulmonary disease (COPD) are more likely to have FHP. It's no surprise that they're fatigued all the time and have low energy levels; it's practically inevitable!

The lack of internal chest area puts pressure on the heart and compresses blood vessels that supply and receive oxygen to and from the heart, as well as restricting breathing capacity. In addition, FHP compressss the distances between the neck and upper thoracic vertebrae, putting pressure on the neck and upper thoracic spine's spinal nerves.

Furthermore, the forward head position restricts the vertebral arteries that transport blood up to the head, reducing blood flow to the face, sections of the brain, and the brainstem, which houses the social-engagement cranial nerves V, VII, IX, X, and XI. When the supply of blood to these cranial nerves is cut off, you look pale, are unable to show spontaneous emotions, and are socially unengaged as one would expect. If these five cranial nerve branches do not get enough blood, they might cease functioning properly and induce chronic stress or dorsal vagal activity.

Breathing problems, minor back discomfort, and discomfort and stiffness in the spine are all typical symptoms of kyphosis. The ear should be positioned just above the midline of your shoulder when seen from the side.

Many people develop a forward head position as they age. In this situation, the ear may be seen moving forward with respect to the shoulder center. You generally have your back hunched, your upper chest is compressed, and your head is no longer supported by your neck. The neck muscles must exert a great deal of effort to keep your head from falling forward.

The more room in the upper chest offered by the Salamander Exercises can help with both the heart and lungs. The nerves that link the spine to the heart, lungs, and visceral organs are relieved of strain when there is less forward head position. The alignment of the cervical vertebrae improves as a result of Salamander Exercises, reducing pressure on vertebral blood vessels and alleviating some discomfort between the shoulders.

You bring your head to the same level as the rest of your spine when you perform the Salamander Exercises. While reptiles and mammals can move their heads in different ways, a salamander's head is much more stationary. It cannot flex, extend, rotate, or side-bend with respect to the first vertebra of the spine. Additionally, it cannot raise its head above the level of other spinal vertebrae.

This exercise is performed with the head in alignment with the spine. The Thoracic may now bend to the side more easily, like a salamander. To alleviate muscle tensions and improve mobility, do side-bending exercises in your thoracic vertebrae.

Your ribs are able to move much more freely and you're able to breathe properly when the thoracic spine is side-bent. The facet joints of the thoracic vertebrae loosen, making it easier for the thoracic spine bend to the side.

There are various modifications to this exercise. You can start one by one depending on whichever feels comfortable doing:

I. Take a seat or stand in a comfortable position. Allow your gaze to shift to the right without rotating your head. Tilt your head to the right, keeping your back straight, such that your right ear is closer to your right shoulder without rising your shoulder to meet it. For thirty to sixty seconds, keep your head in this position. Next, slowly tilt your head back to its original position and gazed ahead. Repeat the process on the other side by looking left with just your eyes then followed by bending your head towards the left hand side before returning both your gaze and head upright after thirty to sixty seconds have passed.

II. Follow the steps in (I), but instead of tilting your head to the left, look to the right. Moving your gaze in the other direction before moving your head should allow you to tilt your head farther to the left; you should be able to twist it even further. Repeat this exercise on both sides for 60 seconds, then do it again on the opposite side.

III. Instead of only bending your neck to the side, bend your whole spine. You'll also need to realign your body position. Get down on all fours, supporting yourself with only the palms of your hands pressed into the ground.

You can place your hands on the floor, but it's preferable to grasp a desktop, a table, the seat of a chair, or the cushion of a sofa. Your head should be in line with the rest of your body. During this exercise, your ears should not be raised higher than or lower than the level of your spine.

To obtain the ideal head posture, slightly raise your head above where you think it should be positioned. Your head should feel lighter than usual. Then lower your head back down to a comfortable position. You'll know if yourHead is too low if you feel tension in your neck or shoulders. Once you've found a good position foryourhead, tiltit sot That yur front right ear moves towardyourright shoulder blades and side-bends tothe rightsimmerly

Use your right hand to balance yourself. Bend simultaneously at the waist and at the back, allowing the curve in your side to extend down your spine and beyond your neck. Maintain this posture for thirty to sixty seconds. Return your spine and head to their original positions after performing all of them on the right side.

Exercises for migraine

The sternocleidomastoid and trapezius muscles produce large rotational movements of the head on the neck, whereas the little suboccipital muscles between the occiput and first two vertebrae of the neck fine-tune these motions. The suboccipital triangle is made up of three of these muscles.

When these deep neck muscles are tensed, they can squeeze the suboccipital nerve and adjacent vertebral arteries inserted in the connective tissue of the suboccipital triangle. This reduces blood flow to the brainstem and five cranial nerves, which are essential for social interaction.

The suboccipital triangle's muscles tighten in a forward head position to keep the chin from sliding onto the chest. If these muscles remain constantly contracted, they will get tighter and tighter, maintaining the forward head posture and restricting blood flow to the brainstem.

Many people with FHP experience headaches in the back of their necks, directly underneath the base of their skulls. This area is where suboccipital muscles are located, and pain here is often caused by pressure on suboccipital nerves. Some individuals who suffer from these headaches report feeling as though they do not have enough nutrients being transported to their heads.

Other symptoms of migraines, in addition to the typical pain, can include fuzzy vision, nausea and vomiting, hypersensitivity to light and sound, fatigue, Aura perception (visual distortions), and vertigo. Additionally, women may suffer from headaches at a specific time during their menstrual cycle.

By focusing on the surface muscles and theirassociated trigger points, you can relieve tension throughout the entire muscle with only a light touch. There is no need to put forth a lot of effort or deeply knead the flesh as you would in traditional massage.

Trigger points are frequently unpleasant to massage deeply or with a lot of force, and this is ineffective. When the body is under a lot of stress, it does not feel secure; as a result, the autonomic nervous system goes into sympathetic activation or dorsal vagal withdrawal mode. This is neither harmful nor wasteful because the body needs time to recover from shock.

I. The indentations on either side of the region where the bridge of your nose meets the ridge of your brows are where your fingers should be positioned. Apply strong pressure to both locations with both index fingers at the same time. For a total of 10 seconds, hold. Then release and repeat the procedure. Touching these pressure points might alleviate headaches caused by eye strain and sinus discomfort or pressure.

II. The gates of consciousness pressure points are located in the hollow spaces between the two vertical cervical muscles at the base of the skull. To find these pressure spots, place your index and middle fingers on both sides of your head with either hand. For 10 seconds, press hard upward while maintaining equal pressure on both sides, then release and repeat. Tension headaches can be relieved by applying strong pressure to these areas.

III. The pressure points at the base of the skull are in parallel hollow spaces between the two vertical neck muscles at the base of the skull. Place your index and middle fingers on the pressure points with either hand. On both sides, apply strong upward pressure for 10 seconds before releasing and repeating. Pressure applied to these areas can reduce tension headaches.

IV. The shoulder well pressure point is located in the center of the soft area between your neck and shoulder. Use one hand to apply strong, circular pressure on this pressure point for 1 minute. Then repeat with other side. By applying firm pressure onto your Shoulder Well Pressure Point, it can help reduce tension in not only your neck and shoulders but also ease discomfort in your necks which often lead to headaches.

Draw circles on the pressure points, and then wait for a nervous system reaction like a sigh or swallow. The discomfort should start to go away within minutes. Use these procedures whenever you need migraine relief.

V. The union valley points are between your thumb and index finger on the web. Begin by pinching this region firmly but not uncomfortably with your opposite hand's thumb and index finger for ten seconds.

Next, for ten seconds at a time, create tiny circles with your thumb in one direction and then the other on this specific pressure point. On your other hand, repeat the process on the union valley point. Pressure point therapy is often said to help lower stress levels in the head and neck area. Tension headaches are commonly linked to high levels of stress.

reflexology is said to relieve headaches, even though it doesn't apply direct pressure to trigger points in the head. Reflexologists exert pressure on specific points of the hands and feet. Reflexology is a calming technique that may assist in relieving tension. This therapeutic technique is based on the belief that different areas of the foot and hand correspond to various organs and systems in the body. By applying pressure to specific points on the hand, it is said to relax and heal corresponding areas of the body.

Exercises for stiff neck

This exercise will increase your range of motion, relieve stiff neck discomfort, and help you avoid migraine headaches as you turn your head.

I. Start by lying down on your stomach. Next, raise your head slightly and cross your arms in front of your chest for support. turning only your head, look over to the right as far as you can comfortably manage. For sixty seconds, stay in that position. Return your gaze to the center. Now turn your head to the left as far as it could comfortably go and hold for sixty seconds.

II. Look up at the ceiling and straighten your back while bending your head backward gently without arching your back. Keep it for five seconds. Move your head down and touch your chest with your chin. Hold the position for five seconds before moving on to the next exercise.

III. Keep your head straight to begin this exercise. Place your right hand on the right side of your temple. Slowly turn your head to the right, pushing and resisting with your hand. Hold the position for five seconds. Repeat on the other side. Repeat ten times.

IV. Slowly raise both of your shoulders while keeping your head straight. Hold the position for five seconds then repeat this process ten times.

V. Put your non-dominant arm in an L-shaped form using your index finger and thumb whilst curling back the other fingers. Place this under your chin, as this will serve as support. With your dominant hand behind your head at the occipital area, lift up and over. This exercise doesn't require much force. Stay in this position for five seconds, and then release slowly while keeping your head in a neutral position.

Generate resistance by placing your hand at the back of your head, just above your neck. Push against your palm for five seconds then release. Next, put pressure on the bridge of your nose and resist with other hand for five seconds followed by slowly pushing against temple while resisting with hand. Repeat these steps on the other side too.

This posture is wonderful for folks who sit at a computer all day and lean back while their heads move forward, putting a lot of strain on the occipital region and restricting blood flow. This might need to be done several times each day, but one round should be enough. Because there is an increase in blood flow to the cranium during this exercise, you may feel lightheaded.

VI. Sit with a straight back, neck, and head. Tilt your chin down to your right shoulder. Use your right hand to pull your head down even more. Put your left hand on the arm of the chair for support. Hold this position for 30 seconds before repeating on the other side three times."

VII. Wearing a towel around your neck, wrap your hands around the ends and gently turn your head back until your eyes are looking up. Apply modest pressure to the towel as you roll your head against it, providing support for your neck. Without holding the stretch, return to the original position. Do ten repetitions in total.

VIII. Place a mat on the floor, lie down flat on your back, and run your fingers through your hair from your neck to scalp. You may need to lift your head slightly off the ground while doing this. Alternatively, you can do this standing up or sitting in a chair.

This massage will help increase blood flow and circulation to your brain. You can run your fingers through your hair ten times for each set, and repeat this until you feel more clear-headed and relaxed neck.

If you have increased your head rotation with these exercises, but your mobility on one side is still limited, the limitation is most likely coming from another muscle, likely the levator scapulae, which is innervated by spinal nerves C3–C5. The strengths of CN XI, the trapezius, and the sternocleidomastoid muscles will not be enough to alleviate this type of stiff neck.

IX. Massaging the levator scapulae is not effective in fixing muscular weakness immediately. The muscular debility will return shortly after you apply pressure to the levator scapulae. It's possible that the under-toned levator scapula is to blame. If you want a longer-lasting benefit, use your fingertips to massage the supraspinatus muscle at the top of the shoulder blade, which will help boost levator scapulae tonus.

Trapezius Exercises

There are always unevenness differences between the fiber groups that make up the upper, middle, and lower trapezius muscles. There is a difference in opinion between the right and left sides as well. The asymmetry of the various components might cause the two shoulders to become out of balance.

Because tension mismatches between the right and left trapezius muscles cause thoracic vertebrae rotations, extensions, flexions, and side-bending, this compromises the chest's internal space.

The imbalance caused by an asymmetrical spine can sometimes put too much pressure on the spinal nerves as they exit these segments. This damage to the organs supplied by those nerves is what we call "referred pain." For example, some spinal nerves from T1 to T4 go to the heart, while others from T5 to T8 connect with the lungs. Other circuits link numerous visceral organs from areas below T9 down through the tailbone.

This exercise not only tones the flaccid trapezius muscle but balances its three sections. It also helps with spine lengthening, respiratory improvement, and correcting forward head position. As a result, you will likely see reduced shoulder and back discomfort. This activity is beneficial to everyone and takes less than a minute to complete--you can see results immediately.

This exercise is best performed after sitting for long periods of time, and should be done regularly. It's already recommended to move around if you frequently work sitting down, so this is an ideal way to integrate physical activity into your daily routine. Each time you perform the exercise, it can improve your breathing and posture, and the benefits will accumulation over time.

This activity is designed to strengthen and stretch the trapezius muscle. It's thought that the muscle is strong enough, so all that's necessary now is nerve activation of flaccid muscle fibers. You're reactivating dormant muscles so they may contribute their fair share of effort. After performing this exercise, you will have a more balanced tone in all of your trapezius muscle fibers.

When you stand or sit, your head should naturally move back and forth, minimizing FHP and enhancing posture.

I. Take a seat on a solid surface, such as the seat of a chair or a bench, and relax. Maintain a forward-facing posture. Fold and cross your arms, softly resting your hands on your elbows. You should quickly rotate your shoulder from one side to the other without pausing or shifting your hips.

Allow your elbows to descend and rest directly in front of your torso throughout the initial segment of the exercise. Rotate your shoulders to the point where your elbows travel from one side to the other. Your arms slide smoothly over your tummy as you swivel your shoulders from side to side.

This exercises targets the higher trapezius muscles. Here are the instructions: Repeat this process three times total. Do not push too hard, and do not stop moving your shoulders-- they should be relaxed and natural throughout the entire movement. Next, with your elbows elevated and in front of your chest at heart level, begin rotating them to one side and then slowly move to the other side.

Repeat three times. Raise your elbows as high as possible comfortably go for the third part, then repeat the exercise. Rotate your elbows from side to side three times. This stimulates the lower trapezius muscle fibers. You may find that your head feels lighter and has shifted back and up, away from the forward head posture once you have completed the exercise.

Someone who does the FHP exercise for the first time usually grows an inch or two taller. If you take a picture of yourself from the side, you will notice that your head is no longer tilted forward like it used to be.

Facial Exercises

This easy and pleasant approach relaxes face muscles and leaves a more natural smile in place by enhancing the function of cranial nerves V and VII. This activity improves skin circulation and restores the expression muscles in the center region of your face, between the edges of your lips and eyes.

Not only does this method improve blood circulation to the skin on your face, which in turn makes you look younger and more restored, but it also encourages you to smile naturally more often. Additionally, it can either raise or lower cheekbones depending on where they sit currently. Before beginning, take a good look at yourself in the mirror and make observations about the skin around your cheekbones. Start with one side of your face before moving onto the other.

Afterwards, see if there is any dissimilarity between the two sides. When you talk or grin, usually the distinctions are visible. Next, do it to the other side until symmetry appears again. The large intestine acupuncture meridian's endpoint is a spot on the face called LI 20 that improves respiration by unclogging your nose. It resides just above where the maxilla and premaxilla--two facial bones--meet."

The two bones mentioned joined together to form a single bone in our species' evolutionary progress. In current anatomy, the maxilla is only regarded as a single bone. If you're struggling to locate The Large Intestine Meridian's terminal, don't worry. It's simple enough to find; just an eighth of an inch to the side of the top of the supra-alar crease (the fold between the cheek and upper lip) at the outer border of your nostril should do it!

The fifth cranial nerve branches innervate the surface of the facial skin, and these touch-sensitive nerve endings are located in an easily found region on your face. If you lightly stroke this area with your finger, it will be more sensitive than the rest of your skin.

I. Gently brush your finger over the surface of your skin at acupuncture point LI 20. Sink your fingertip into the skin and slide it up and down to see which direction offers more resistance. Push gently into this stiffness until you reach a stopping point. Hold that position and wait for the tension to release. To find out which way has increased resistance, slide the skin toward the center line of your face or outward toward the side.

Stop. Softly push. Hold your breath and wait for the release. The seventh cranial nerve's branches innervate the facial muscles. Just below the epidermis, there are two face muscle layers. Gently dip your fingers into these muscular layers beneath the skin simultaneously."

The first muscle layer should be pushed against your fingers. You can move these layers of muscles by being careful not to push too hard, and if you feel what is happening under your skin; First, create circular motions. This can help in moving the muscle and skin layers. Some resistance may be felt while moving the skin in one direction as it becomes difficult to move around in circles.

Begin to press gently in that direction and hold until a sigh or swallow signifies release. The following time you repeat this, push a little harder. The adhesion of the deeper muscles to the upper layer of muscles has now occurred. With this exercise, all layers may be slid together over the bone's surface. Massaging on the periosteum's surface has a significant impact on the autonomic nervous system.

At Large Intestine 20 (LI 20), press softly but hard enough to reach the bone's surface. Allow your fingertip to slide from side to side on the bone's surface, then apply gentle pressure to the bone and wait for a release, which is usually either a sigh or a swallow.

The nerves to the skin and muscles of the face are stimulated by massaging cranial nerves V and VII. Wrinkles will not disappear completely, butcrow's feet, laugh lines, and wrinkles caused by sun damage lessen. There is no risk for negative side effects like scarring.

We should be able tochange and control our facial expressions to show a range of emotions depending on the situation. This is important for how we communicate nonverbally with others, and this activity can help strengthen that skill. These variations in skin and facial muscle tension subsequently send feedback to the brain via cranial nerves V and VII's afferent pathways, providing you with instant subconscious knowledge about how others are feeling.

If you want people to see that you empathy, you must have facial expressions that match. Unfortunately, a lot of us get stuck making the same emotional and consequent physical face for years. Our facial muscles then sag and pulled down by gravity, resulting in wrinkles and a double chin.

If a person continues to feel the same emotional state over time and does not relaxing their muscles, these lines will deepen. Activating CN V through stroking the skin decreases tension for all facial muscles.

The first facial exercise is not the only one. This focuses on your eyes. In many ways, the second exercise is identical to the first. Acupuncture point B2 can be found in the inner corner of the brow, where your eyebrows begin. When people are exhausted, they frequently massage this region while focusing on it consciously. Self-soothing entails massaging both skin and muscle tissue around the face.

Touch B2 with your thumb or one finger. Move down the different layers of the skin, two layers of muscles, and the periosteum starting at B2. The orbicularis oculi muscle, a thin, flat muscle that borders the eye's entrance, is likewise affected by this location. The eyes, which are said to be the soul's mirror, are often referred to as such. The muscle may be excessively tense, causing the eye to close somewhat, or it can be undertoneed, causing the eye to open too widely before you start working on B2.

If you follow these steps, you will find it easier to maintain eye contact with others and they may see you in a better light. First, focus on making balance between looking outwards and inwards. By doing so, you will be able to see other people more clearly which makes it less daunting for them approach you.

II. Find the spot on the inner corner of your brow that is more sensitive than the rest of your brow. To begin, softly brush the skin with your fingers a few times. Allow your fingertip to rest lightly on the skin at point B2 and keep it there until you feel a release in the form of a sigh or a swallow. Next, gently press down on the layer of facial muscles.

The orbicularis oculi is a flat, circular muscle that goes around the eye and connects to the face's bones. To find the tension point, allow your skin to stick to your finger then make small circles with light pressure. You should feel resistance in one direction. Stay on this spot until you release a sigh or swallow reflexively. Then, dig deeper until you reach the bone's surface.

Rub your hands together a few times. Then keep your hand on the bone and wait for it to pop free. Closing the eyelids into squints if the orbicularis oculi muscle is excessively tight should open the eye more normally. If the eye was previously too wide, this technique should help to narrow it somewhat while still leaving it open.

The massage's purpose is to leave you with a smile on your lips and a sparkle in your eyes.

Facial Massage

This exercise will stimulate the vagus nerve by moving the facial muscles. You'll need a set of therapeutic yoga balls for this treatment. If you don't have access to a set, you may do the activity with your index fingers instead. This also induces a relaxation response while easing your facial muscles and making them more expressive.

I. Locate the TMJ area by feeling for where the maxilla and mandible meet, then use the yoga balls to massage in an up-and-back direction towards your ears. You don't need to apply pressure on or near your teeth. Keep the yoga tone-up balls at this location and slowly open and close your mouth. You can also try to move the lower jaw forward whilst you twist the yoga tone-up balls in place. Jars your jaw from side to side as you do this exercise. This will help stimulate the pterygoid muscle, which is the depressor muscle of the mouth. These muscles on each side of the jaw play an important role in TMJ and mandible joint movements.

II. The elevator labial superior muscles, located on either side of your nose, are another key target during this exercise. If you have a set of therapeutic yoga balls available, place them on these muscles and try to traction them with the side of the ball or fingers. As you press back with your fingers, let them hang behind the muscle. Whilst you apply pressure, try to twist the balls in place. This technique is great for clearing your sinuses.

III. Grab one of the therapeutic yoga balls and place it between your eyebrows for an additional approach to employ while using these balls. Twist the ball in place while applying slight pressure. Again, let your head lean forward while the ball is pushing backward. This helps to take off the tension in that muscle, which is often used in expressions of worry.

IV. Place the two yoga therapeutic balls one on each side of your temporalis, against your temples. You might alternatively use your index fingers to do this. Twist the balls in place while applying pressure with your fingertips at the sides of your eyes. Pluck the skin at the temporalis if you're using your hands. Open and close the jaw when doing this exercise.

This series of facial massages can help you put your best face forward as you move through life.

Exercises to increase social engagement.

The purpose of this exercise is to improve social interactions by repositioning the first and second cervical vertebras, C1 and C2. This will increase mobility in the neck and spine while also improving blood flow to the brainstem. The ventral branch of the vagus nerve may also see benefits from this cranial nerves exercise.

This easy two-minute exercise will strengthen your neck muscles and improve your range of motion. Gently tilt your head to the right, then back to the center. Next, turn your head to the left side. Finally, return to looking straight ahead again. When you have better neck mobility, more blood flow goes to the brainstem. This increased function of the vagus nerve's ventral branch helps you detect changes.

I. You should begin by performing the exercise on your back for the first several times. After you've gotten used to it, you may carry out the activity while sitting in a chair, standing, or lying down on your back. Intertwine the fingers of one hand with those of the other while resting comfortably on your back.

Interlace your fingers behind your head, resting the weight of your skull on top of them. With your emails, feel the solidity of your skull as well as the bones in your fingers touching the back of it. If you have tightness in one shoulder and can't put both hands behind comfortably, use just one hand with its fingers and palm flush against both sides at the back of your head.

Simply look to the right as far as you can without moving your head. Simply move your eyes rather than turning your head. Continue to look to the right. You may swallow, yawn, or exhale after a brief amount of time, up to thirty seconds. This is due to the autonomic nervous system's relaxation.

After you inhale, exhale normally. But when you sigh, take a second exhalation on top of the first one. Follow this by another normal exhalation. Next, return your gaze to a straight-ahead position and keep your hands where they are. Then fix your gaze steadily on a spot to the left until you sigh, yawn or swallow. Once you've completed the exercise, go ahead and stand up or sit down as desired."

When you sit up or stand, you may feel dizzy due to the decrease in blood pressure from lying down. This is normal.

The following method, on the other hand, needs less than five minutes and only requires minimal physical effort. It may be used on oneself or others. You must stimulate reflexes in the nerves in loose connective tissue beneath the skin at the base of the skull to utilize this technique to increase social interaction.

II. This method is easiest to learn when you are lying on your stomach, as you will be able to see your fingers more easily. Start by feeling the occipital bone at the back of your head. Gently press near the base of the head on one side to get a sense of its firmness. Then test the skin's "slide-ability" on one side of the occiput by sliding it to the right over the bone.

Allow the skin to swing back and forth a few times. When it reaches toward you, slowly press your thumb into it towards the center of its pattern. Then wait for it to come back to where you started. After that, move the skin to the other side, let go of it, and have it return to its original position. Make a mental note of which region had more resistance. To assist relieve tension, move the skin in the direction where there was most resistance was felt.

Once you hit the first sign of resistance, slowly back off and be prepared to stop. It may have barely moved an eighth of an inch--stop there and stay put. Continue to feel slight resistance as you do nothing but sigh or swallow; eventually, the skin's tension will give way as it relaxes.

Test the skin's movement in both directions. If it meets resistance or feels peculiar, check the other side for reference. The vagus nerve should be fully operational. increased flexibility should also be felt when turning the head from side to side..

Once you are confident with the above exercise, you should try following this one:

III. Place your index finger on the back of your head, at the base, behind your ear. As mentioned before, test how easily the skin slides over the bone. It should be more flexible in one direction than it is in another. Place your opposite hand's index finger at the top of your neck on that same side.

If you're pushing and don't feel any resistance from the muscles, increase the pressure. Test how far you can move your skin over the muscles at the top of your neck with one finger. The other finger should slide easily over your skull now. When you've finished the exercise, lighten up on the pressure.

Allow your two fingers to move in opposite directions across the skin until you feel resistance. Stop there and maintain that little strain; wait for a sigh or a swallow. After releasing your fingertips, allow the skin to return to its natural position.

The process should be repeated on the skin of the other side of the skull and neck before testing the vagus nerve again. If it is now fully functional, there will be more flexibility when rotating the head to left and right.

Practices for Post-traumatic stress disorder

PTSD (post-traumatic stress disorder) is a frequent diagnosis. After a traumatic experience, you should be able to return to a state of social engagement if you have a strong autonomic nervous system.

Unfortunately, not all individuals recover. Everyone has traumatic and unpleasant events in their lives, yet people react differently to similar experiences. On the one hand, some can swiftly overcome them, regain their equilibrium and social connection, and move on with their life.

On the contrary, what happens to other people alters them in different ways that can have long-lasting and even incapacitating consequences. These may follow the individual for the rest of their life.

Many people who are depressed struggle with dorsal vagal activation. Therapists usually choose to focus on the trauma itself instead of the psychophysiological response that came after the event while treating post-traumatic stress disorder. recounting what happened and telling someone else about it is one way to relieve post-traumatic stress, but it is not always effective because reliving the event can retraumatize individuals.

The first step in treating PTSD is to get people out of a state of activity in their spinal sympathetic circuit or dorsal vagal nerve and back into social engagement. The second stage is to keep them socially engaged by repeating the procedure as needed. The following activities are all useful techniques for persons with PTSD, especially those that aim to improve their social interaction skills.

Get rid of stress cortisol by moving your body. Rub your hands together quickly and touch your face, neck, upper chest, arms, and legs to stimulate your social nerve system. You can also relieve tension by doing physically secure and grounding activities like walking or shaking your arms and legs. If you have a friend, spouse, or pet that you love spending time with, turn to them for support.

To begin, you may need to make eye contact with someone you trust or call them and listen to their voice. Imagine a cherished animal or companion to re-establish a sense of connection. Accepting immobility with safety allows you to obtain the benefits of the relaxation response.

The polyvagal theory in action might assist you feel more free in your body and mind when you experience anxiety, panic, or sadness. Focus on the present moment and select an essential oil with a pleasant scent connection or sensation to use your sense of smell. Feelings may be expressed through words, writing, art, or movement.

Consider breathing as a fine-tuning technique for nerve system management. Engage in a mindfulness-based practice such as meditation or yoga therapy. Allow yourself to have fun and be creative by giving yourself permission. Concentrate on the good by appreciating nature's beauty around you.

Abdominal Massage

This massage should only take a few minutes, and it can be done at home. Make sure you do this exercise on an empty stomach, a few hours after eating. Start carefully and observe how your body reacts.

I. Lie back on a soft floor mat or a comfy bed. Put your hand just below your sternum (breastbone). Moving your hand down toward your abdomen, make soft downward stroking movements. For a few minutes, run one hand over the other in a reverse bike-pedaling motion.

Finish with a few circular motions on your abdomen with your fingertips. Begin by rubbing the sides of your stomach and working your way closer to the middle. Continue going deeper, maintaining a firm yet pleasant level of pressure. Continue massaging your belly for several minutes at the end of your session. Toward the end, spend a few moments in a comfortable seated two-knee spinal twist posture.

This restorative yoga pose can help improve your digestion and encourage an opening in the fascia and diaphragm, which will deepen your breath and generate an anti-inflammatory relaxation response.

Begin by breathing into your legs as you press your lower back to the floor or bed. Take a few deep breaths while your lower back opens up. Once you've taken in enough air, bend your knees and clench your abdominal muscles before exhaling and extending your arms out to the side with palms facing down.

On a deep inhale, raise your heels a little higher than your knees. As you exhale, smoothly lower both legs to the left until they are close to the floor. Your knees should be at hip level and feet pressing against each other. Rest in this position for thirty seconds up to one minute. Continue to take slow, deep breaths as you twist from side to side, moving your breath with you.

II. This core exercise necessitates the use of a tiny core ball. Face the floor and lie down, placing the ball beneath your belly. Inhale deeply and hold your breath while making tension in your body with inhales. Try to keep the core ball from sinking into the skin by creating tension while holding your breath. This will strengthen your core. After a few moments, exhale and allow the ball to sink into your skin and abdomen..

Whilst you hold your breath and create tension, all your muscles in the abdomen are contracted. You can feel the outer layers of the muscles and notice the tension in them. Repeat this a couple of times, and you should notice that after you exhale, the ribcage will encircle the ball as the ball enters the abdomen.

III. If you have experienced bloating or intestinal disorders such as Crohn's disease or colitis, this exercise may provide some relief. However, if you have had surgery in the past - especially hernia repair that included abdominal mesh - it is best to avoid this movement. Additionally, those who lack flexibility may find it difficult to do; though people familiar with yoga should be able to complete the stretch without issue.

This practice will help with blood circulation in the abdominal region, which can be beneficial for menstruating women. Blood flow in the stomach is necessary for everyone, though. The small intestine, in particular, is targeted by this exercise. A softball is required for this activity; a hard medicine ball may also be used. Because softer balls would not put pressure on your abdomen, they will not suffice.

Lie on your back on a mat and place the softball to the left of your hip, so that blood flow can improve at the descending colon. However, eventually you should repeat this exercise on the right side as well. To start, bring your left leg up and then grab hold of it with both hands near the knee area while also pulling it towards your face.

Make a fist with your arm bent and place it behind your head. This is done while standing or sitting on the floor. Start out with a small squeeze. You'll need to be able to breathe comfortably while performing this exercise, yet as you push the ball inwards, breathing may become more difficult. Your ball should sink into your belly. As you exhale, allow your feet to move inwards while increasing pressure on the ball with each breath. The softball might shift about as you work, so feel free to move it about if this occurs.

Exhale, then stay on one side for three to four breaths. Try to keep your breath for a few seconds before inhaling again to focus the softball's pressure in the region. You may apply the same technique on both sides and push the ball higher up your abdomen, just below your rib cage, to target the small intestine.

Insert the softball into the abdominal cavity without putting pressure on the ribs. You can press around the belly button by moving the ball or lifting both of your feet as you pull further up. Continue this exercise for 15-20 minutes, until you've gone around the entire abdominal area.

Exercise for a hiatal hernia

A hiatal hernia can be treated with an osteopathic visceral-massage technique that is shown below. It's a simple self-help exercise that delivers remarkable results. A basic osteopathic treatment is to pull the stomach down to elongate and relax the esophagus. Asthma, pulmonary fibrosis, and shortness of breath may all be relieved by this procedure. On the left side of the abdomen, directly beneath the rib cage is the stomach.

I. Place your fingertips of one hand on the top of where you believe the stomach to be. Although the tummy is soft, it is identifiable. If you gently explore the abdominal muscles with your fingertips, you should be able to feel the stomach. All you need to do is feel what's above the stomach's top layer.

The top of the stomach should never be touched. This approach should not cause any discomfort; if it does, you should stop immediately. Slowly draw it down to your feet until you feel resistance, which is usually after about a half-inch to an inch of pulling. Hold it there until the esophagus releases with only a little resistance at that point.

There's no need to push your stomach down when trying to lengthen your esophagus. Just put your fingers on the top of your stomach and the nerves will extend, which in turn makes the inhalation easier.

The act of breathing in, holding one's breath and then exhaling is commonly accompanied by a deep sigh or a swallow. The muscular resistance to the stomach being dragged down appears to fade at this time. You can breathe more easily and fully right now.

The stomach can slide downwards into a lower position in the belly because to a relaxed esophagus, which provides it more area to move. This also allows the diaphragm to glide freely up and down across the outside surface of the esophagus, routinely travelling over

When you practice this technique, your respiration will become noticeably slower and deeper. With each breath, more air will be exchanged. Not only can this be a temporary alternative to surgery for hiatal hernia, but it can also help with other conditions like COPD and difficulty breathing.

Ear Exercises

Although you may not believe your ears can be stiff, they might get somewhat uncomfortable if you haven't achieved a vagal tone. The auricular branches of the vagus nerve originate in the ear and are known as such. Try closing your eyes while evaluating whether or not you're in a vagal tone.

One ear may be a little tighter than the other on occasion. When you pull, does one of your ears seem more soft or rigid? Take notice of whether you can move it up and down and how that feels. After testing for vagal tone using your ear, you may proceed with this exercise. You may check back with this technique after doing the exercise to see if your ears are less tight.

I. To clear your ear, you must first access the hollow area of your ear above the ridge near to your ear canal. Gently move your finger along the hollow above the ridge with a circular motion. At this location, you are not required to apply any great pressure; rather, consider rotating the skin in circles.

For this exercise, you won't need to apply much pressure. You may notice changes in your breathing while doing it - such as sighing or swallowing. Once you're done with one side, repeat the process on the other ear. While some people feel a sense of calmness after doing it, that's not required.

When one ear is being massaged, you may feel such physical symptoms while the other ear remains unaffected. There is no specific time limit for this exercise. Feel free to spend as much time as you wish on it.

The vagus nerve can be accessed at the ear but from a different area. Here is how:

II. The vagus nerve may also be stimulated at the back of your ear canal, which is a more natural approach. To massage the region, follow the same technique: press firmly towards the back of your head while making small circles with your index finger. Because there isn't any pressing to do here, simply move the skin in circular motions instead

The head travels in a circular motion, providing sensory data to your nerve system. In this case, applying additional force is ineffective. After completing one side, repeat the process on the other ear.

While massaging, you may find that one side is easier to manipulate than the other. This will help confirm that you are not in a vagal tone. It is crucial to be aware of these small distinctions while massaging. There is also no time limit for this method, so you can continue as long as desired.

III. The test technique mentioned previously can not only be used to check the status of your vagus nerve, but it can also act as a means of stimulation. To do this, apply pressure for a longer period of time than you did during the initial test.

Take your ear and gently stretch it. This focuses on stretching the entire ear without applying too much force. If you have temporomandibular (TMJ) problems, this is a great way to stretch your ear. The sliding connection between your jawbone and skull is referred to as this region. On each side of the jaw, TMJ issues can be caused by injury to teeth, bruxism, poor posture, stress, or arthritis.

If you're seeking relief from stress headaches, this exercise might do the trick. Gently pull your ear away from your skull as you perform the activity. This sends messages to your nervous system that elicits a calming response.

Start on one ear and do the other side. It's possible that you feel discomfort in one ear, but not the other. If this is the case, don't practice this exercise on the painful side since it will be ineffective.

IV. Slide your head gently upwards from the bottom of your hairline, taking care to stretch skin behind your ear upward. Stretching the skin behind your ear upwards is a must. You should only stretch the skin for a few moments at a time without adding pressure. This transmits information via your nerves to your brain.

This helps your brain to realize that the muscles in that area can move, in turn releasing that area. Once you are done pulling the skin up, take the same area and pull it down towards your neck and away from the top of your head. Hold the stretch in both directions. Do the same technique but pull towards the back of your head. Repeat the same technique to the other side.

As with the other ear exercises, there is no specified duration for which you must continue performing this exercise. One movement may appear to be simpler than the others on one side. This is quite normal, and it's advised that you repeat the drill in the direction where your skin flows more freely since it is more productive and efficient.

Feel free to check for tightness in your ears after performing these procedures, as described above. These routines may help you relax around the neck and jaw. When breathing is easier through the sinuses, your eyes might feel softer. You can use this approach to relieve sudden stress and anxiety right now.

Visceral Massage

Massaging the organs below your diaphragm can help stimulate the vagus nerve. You require a core ball and a yoga block for this exercise.

I. Lie down on the yoga block with your head against the side of your abdomen and the core ball beneath your abdomen. This exercise might be more beneficial to you if you expose your skin, so take off your shirt or tuck it up for this activity.

The core ball should be inserted between your right ribs as far as it will go. Begin by moving to one side, allowing your abdomen to slide over the core ball. While your hand is positioned above this region, fatty tissue and visceral organs should be on the core ball in order for it to work properly. Your hand has now become a heavy weight on your stomach.

The deep breathing technique mentioned earlier should be utilized during this process. As you breathe, you should take note of your stomach rising and falling. With time, as this exercise starts working, sounds signifying digestion will start being heard emanating from your gut--a certain indication that the vagus nerve has been sufficiently stimulated.

This technique helps to move gas down the sigmoid area of the intestines and out when laying down on the left. When turning to your right, digested food is encouraged to move through the intestines. Allow a few minutes on each side for this exercise.

Neck Massage

Using a core ball against the neck exerts pressure which in turn stimulates your vagus nerve. This exercise can activate the relaxation response.

I. Against the side of your neck, below your ears, place the core ball. Then, spin the ball around your neck ensuring that you roll it against soft tissue lining the inside of your neck. The movement should be fluid as if you're shaving off a beard but with the core ball instead of a blade; from one ear to another.

The core ball is designed to target the larynx and trachea- two sensitive areas located in the front of the neck. As you roll across these area, release pressure slightly before continuing on to massage deeper muscle layers at each side of your neck.

The core ball applies pressure to the carotid artery when you massage the lateral muscles of the neck, which innervates the vagus nerve. This will help reduce heart rate and breathing pace, therefore inducing relaxation.

The benefits of horseback riding may be enjoyed for a longer period of time if you maintain your neck in the correct position. You should practice this exercise for a couple of minutes while going from one side to the other several times. When you remove the core ball, you should notice an increase in heat throughout your neck.

After a few moments, your facial muscles should feel as if they are relaxing. The vagus response induced by this practice also affects the facial muscles, head, and neck. After this exercise, you may notice that your hearing and eyesight have improved.

Rib Cage Massage

For this yoga exercise, you will need a block and small ball to help stimulate the vagus nerve through its connections at the diaphragm and lungs.

I. Put your head on a yoga block and the core ball beneath your ribcage, then lie on one side. The core ball must be positioned between the armpit and the first ribs for this exercise to work. Take your other hand and place it over the rib cage. This step requires you to have some internal rotation on that shoulder, but if you struggle with this, place a pillow on that side and let your arm hang down instead.

By still providing pressure to the side, this will place your arm on top of the ribcage. Inhale and hold your breath while contracting your muscles in the ribcage--it may seem as if you're trying to cough, but you're not. Exhale and allow your breath exit your body.

Relax until you feel the need to take a breath, then inhale deeply and hold your breath. As you breathe in during this exercise, expanding your ribs should make it easier to air into your lungs. This enables you focus on feeling your heartbeat. Additionally, this breathing technique is soothing for the nervous system as it Awakens The Vagus Nerve– one of the longest nerves in the body that starts from stem of brain all way down to our abdomen!

II. For this exercise, you will need the small core ball and yoga block from before. Lay on your stomach with the ball placed under your sternum and without the yoga block. Your arms should be crossed over and placed under your head. This pose activates the heart's natural pacemaker, known as to laymen as the sinoatrial node."

Inhale deeply and hold your breath as if you are coughing. release the breath when you feel the urge to breathe again. If anxiety is commonplace for you, aim to repeat this exercise ten to twenty minutes. Doing so will hopefully lower your stress response and make you feel calmer overall.

Breathing immobilization technique

You may utilize this method to combat fatigue or tiredness throughout the day, or if it's past five o'clock in the afternoon and you need some energy to get through the day.

I. To do this breath work, inhale deeply and hold the breath in your lower stomach. Tension should form in your ribcage. Use your fingers to tap on various spots of your trunk while continuing to breathe through pursed lips. Keep tapping until you need to take another breath. By doing this, you are stimulating sympathetic fibers throughout Trunk including those around your heart and lungs

Once you can't hold your breath anymore, exhale and start the process over again. If you have a close friend nearby, they may be able to help by tapping on your back--an area that's difficult to reach by yourself.

This activity may startle you with how long you can hold your breath. By doing this, we are slowly increasing our threshold and resistance in the nervous system. Even though it isn't necessarily a 'relaxing' exercise, it helps us focus because of the repetitiveness of the movement.

Tongue Exercises

I. If you have the ability, look into a mirror while standing up. Move your tongue around in your mouth without letting it go. Try to brush all of your teeth with your tongue. You may observe both the position of your tongue inside your mouth and the direction it is going while looking through the mirror, allowing you to lead it with your index finger.

Make sure your tongue reaches into the inside of your cheeks while you push forward. Breathe through your nose as you perform this exercise. Begin with three to five circles in each direction for a few weeks, then progress to ten circles in each direction. This may be done three to five times a day.

The Acupuncture mats.

Acupressure mats feature hundreds of plastic nubs that apply pressure to the back's acupressure points. Acupressure pillows are also available to use on the neck, head, hands, and feet. Acupressure mats are designed to simulate the benefits of acupressure massage. Acupressure is a method for releasing stopped energy in the body by applying pressure to specific points on the body with your fingers. The technique for stimulating the vagus nerve is comparable to acupuncture.

Acupressure mats are now being utilized by a lot of people to treat back discomfort and headaches. They work by stimulating pressure points along the body's meridians. The difference is that acupressure mats stimulate many acupressure points indiscriminately, whereas professional acupressure or acupuncture treatments target certain acupoints.

It may take some time for your body to adjust to the acupressure mat. The spikes might cause discomfort or pain for several minutes before your body gets used to it. For best results, use the mat for ten to twenty minutes each day. Remember to breathe and intentionally relax your entire body while using the mat..

I. Choose a surface on which to place the mat. You may either lie down on the ground or on a soft surface like a sofa or a yoga mat. The more pressure that the acupoints can apply, the harder the surface should be. You might wish to start with a softer surface and then progress to a harder one over time. Some prefer to sit on it while others choose to put it on a chair instead.

Initially, sit or lie on the mat with an article of clothing between you and the spikes to get accustomed to them. You may eventually choose to forgo this layer. Be sure to distribute your weight evenly and lower yourself slowly onto the mat as too much pressure at once can be uncomfortable.

If you fidget or move too much while using the mat, it'll cause your skin to scratch. If this method works for you, do this exercise regularly because it takes a little time to get used to an acupressure mat. Also, people have said they see more benefits when they use it regularly. You can purchase one online or at a sports store nearby.

Foam Roller Exercises

The thin layer of connective tissue that Fascia is integral to the proper function and alignment of your muscles and organs. Collagen, a protein molecule made up of three helixes linked together, gives fascia its strength. It develops in response to mechanical stressors such as collisions or Single Nucleotide Polymorphisms.

Each muscle fiber contains a ground substance that is made up of individual collagen molecules, which form the extracellular matrix (ECM). The ECM reduces friction when individual muscles fibers move against one another. When tissue is warmed and handled on a regular basis, the ECM becomes more gel-like, reducing friction and making movement between fibers easier.

Inactive muscle fibers cause the collagen molecules in the extracellular matrix to bond together, which then restricts the ability of other fibers to slide against one another.

Adhesions may restrict a muscle's ability to extend and facilitate motion at a joint. Scar tissue is an example of how the ECM's collagen binds together to assist in the recovery of a tissue following injury. When scar tissue forms, it restricts the tissue's movement through its normal range of motion, occasionally affecting joint function.

Collagen is formed parallel to muscle fibers during natural movement and exercise in order to provide structure and flexibility, making the tissue more resilient and prone to strain injuries. Collagen production may be aided by strength-training activities performed in a variety of directions.

The best results come when a person rhythmically applies tension to their muscles and connective tissue with a foam roller. This process helps break up adhesions and restructure muscle tissue so it can function properly.

The rolling action eliminates friction, hydrates, and repairs the tissues of your body as you glide over the roller. This compressed technique unblocks trapped energy, wrings out pollutants, and reduces scar tissue by compressing tissue. When moderate pressure is applied to your fascia and skin by a foam roller, pressure receptors in your fascia and skin are activated. The signal is sent via the vagus nerve to your vagus nerve.

The vagus nerve has branches that extend to all parts of the body, including the heart. When these pressure receptors are stimulated, it slows the heart rate and relaxes you. Massage studies have shown this effect, but there is no reason to believe that self-massage with a foam roller would not have the same impact. As your heart rate lowers, your hormones begin to respond to signals sent from the pressure receptors.

Melatonin controls the release of neurotransmitters and hormones, which are responsible for your moods. Cortisol decreases while serotonin and dopamine, feel-good chemicals in the brain, increase as a result of stress. If you get massages on a regular basis, the hormonal effect lasts longer, and that is one of the benefits of foam rolling using foam rollers at home: you may do it whenever you want. Daily home foam rolling might provide a moderate amount of emotional boost similar to a low dose of antidepressants, providing long-term relief to get you through each day.

Another benefit of foam rolling, according to fascia researchers, is that it may help relieve unpleasant feelings. When you are tense, terrified, or angry, your muscles tighten up. If the emotions are only momentary and last for a few hours or a day, the physical strain will lessen.

When you are constantly stressed, your muscles never get a chance to relax. This causes the fascia (a layer that surrounds the muscle) to thicken and tighten over time.

By stimulating the nerve endings in the fascia, which sends messages to the brain, self-myofascial release (SMR) can help buried emotions rise to the surface. Along with physical discomfort and stress, this process is said to assist in their release. Depending on the techniques you choose, foam rolling can be used for self-massage, stretching, rehabilitation, or even as a workout.

By rolling on a foam roller, you can not only reduce pain or soreness caused by inactivity or exercise, but also develop strong and flexible muscles. In addition, foam rolling provides a comprehensive reboot of your system.

Other physical benefits of foam rolling including improved circulation, improved posture, lymphatic drainage, reduced inflammation, improved digestion, core stabilization, and strengthening.

When first using a foam roller, you will always feel some level of discomfort. It is also important to know that the density of different foam rollers varies. Therefore, if you are new to this or prefer softer pressure, it is best fo find a gentler option. With time and practice, it should begin feeling good on your body.

If you have any medical issues, injuries, or are pregnant, speak with your doctor first. If this seems like a good fit for you, use it every day if that's what you prefer; alternatively, combine it in with anything else you enjoy doing, such as completing your yoga session with a few foam rolling exercises from the list below.

Every once in a while, I suggest going for a walk as part of your training and health routine. For achieving long-term, visible results, consistency is crucial. While many individuals think that stretching should be done after exercise to prepare their bodies for activity, it's preferable to do it before.

In addition, rolling on the ground can help with any pain. If you use a foam roller for myofascial release during your warm-up, it will not only loosen tension but also increase heat in muscle and fascia without tiring you out. It is crucial to only utilize the foam roller for a short time during a warm-up so that tissue temperature rises and tension decreases.

If you stay on a foam roller for an extensive amount of time, it could anaesthetize the muscle and reduce its power to contract during exercise. It's wiser to use the foam roller at nightfall as part of your relaxation routine so that you can de-stress. Internal muscle temperature actually rises when using a foam roller.

When you use a foam roller on your muscles and connective tissue, friction is generated between the roller and the muscle. Because of the higher heat, the tissue becomes more gel-like, making it more malleable. Tissue that is easier to extend after being more extensible enables adjacent joints to achieve full range of motion.

Foam rolling can be a crucial component of warming up before a workout, but in order to experience the best results keep the pressure on each muscle group ranged from two minutes or less. The majority of people nowadays spend hours upon hours slumped over electronic devices. Even if you can only manage to squeeze out five minutes for yourself, it will make an impactful difference.

The ideal way to use a foam roller is to first reduce tissue tension, then make multidirectional movements to help the tissue adapt to the new length while maintaining joint function. Foam rolling has several benefits and is an excellent method for integrating mind and body health approaches.

Try the following exercises on a foam roller to stimulate your vagus nerve:

I. Sit down with your legs spread out in front of you and the foam roller beneath your calves. Using your arms and wrists, roll the foam roller up and down as your calf muscles move up and down on top of it. It's also possible to make it more intense by crossing your legs while you roll up and down.

II. Kneel on your hands and knees with the foam roller underneath your shins. Raise your knees off the ground, draw them up towards your hands, and then return to your position.

III. Sit on the floor with a foam roller placed beneath your knees and your legs extended out in front of you. Gently roll from the back of your knee until you reach your buttocks, focusing on one hamstring at a time. You can target specific muscles by crossing one leg over the other as you complete this exercise.

IV. Position the foam roller underneath your quads and assume a forearm plank posture, lying face down. Use your arms or forearms to move your body up and down the length of your quad muscles, from the front of your hips to the top of your knees.

V. Place your feet flat on the floor and sit on the foam roller. As you semi-recline backward, your hands should also be on the floor. Roll your butt down and up over the foam roller with your arms and legs. By bending your body slightly to one side, you may emphasize the other.

VI. Sit down on your back with your knees bent, cradling your head in your hands, with the foam roller across your shoulder blades. Lift your hips off the floor and make use of your legs to roll your body down and up on the foam roller. Let go of your upper body and let your spine stretch back over the foam roller to maximize stretching at each vertebra.

VII. Use a bigger foam roller for this so that it can run the full length of your spine. Lay down on the roller with your feet flat against the floor and your knees bent. Reach both arms overhead and back towards the floor, holding whatever rod you are using. Return to start after 10 seconds.

VIII. Position the foam roller underneath your armpit and latissimus dorsi (or rear shoulder) then lie on your side with your arm outstretched in front of you or up above your head. Next, use your legs to roll up and down on top of the foam roller.

IX. To massage your bicep with a foam roller, start by lying on your side with your arm extended out to the side. Place the foam roller underneath your bicep, and then cross your feet over and place one of them on top of the other thigh for stability. Use both feet and thighs to slowly roll back-and-forth over the foam roller.

X. Turn your body to the side and again place the foam roller on your armpit. This will massage your triceps. With your feet planted on the floor, roll the foam roller over the area to massage it.

XI. Keep your hands beneath your shoulders and the foam roller under your neck to make it seem like a pillow. While keeping your arms crossed on your chest, tilt your head from side to side.

Quick Vagus nerve reset.

This exercise may be done anywhere, at any time, and requires no equipment. You can either sit or stand while performing this activity.

I. Cover your eyes with your hands. Cover your ears with your thumbs to block distractions that may excite your brain. Hum as you inhale and exhale. This tells your brain that you are secure, and this is where the vagus nerve stimulation kicks in. You'd be combining breathing and humming, two of the most simple yet effective ways to activate your vagus nerve.

II. Another easy way to help stimulate your vagus nerve is by massaging the Sternocleidomastoid (SCM) on both sides of your neck. This muscle runs from behind your ears down to upper part of the chest and can be found easily since it's superficial. If you have trouble finding it, try blatantly moving your head from side to side until you feel the contractions in that area.

Take your hand and pinch along the SCM, starting at the top and working your way down. Some regions may be more difficult to massage than others. This process should not be unpleasant; if it is, you should apply less pressure. The objective of this method is to relieve tension and stimulate the vagus nerve. You may spend a little money on each side before moving on to the other side. For optimum results, repeat this technique at least three times a day every day for three weeks.

The wall stretches.

Find a wall you can use for this exercise.

I. Raise your arms and place them on the wall with the elbows facing the wall. You may also rest your head against the wall if you like. Inhale through your nose and exhale through your mouth as you arch your back and protrude your bottom. On both sides of your body, from armpit to armpit, and from back to buttocks, you should feel a stretch.

II. To do this exercise, you can rest one arm at a time against the wall and apply the same technique to each side separately. Stay in this position for thirty seconds to a minute before shaking it off with some jogging on the spot. This helps release any stressful energy stored in your body and stimulating your vagus nerve. You can repeat this three to four times per day or more if desired.

III. If you already do yoga, you can do this exercise on the floor instead of against a wall. Use both hands at once or one at a time. You can use it to finish off a stretching exercise after a workout, or do it during your nine-to-five job.

This is particularly helpful if you work at a desk and may help to reset your posture and release tension.

Jaw Massage

These exercises are specifically intended for people suffering from TMJ dysfunction or bruxism, commonly known as jaw clenching or teeth grinding. If you clench or grind your teeth, especially at night, you may have bruxism. This condition usually results from anxiety and stress, but can cause headaches, facial pain, or damage to your teeth. To do some of the exercises below, gather a yoga block and set of therapeutic yoga balls before beginning.

I. Place the therapeutic balls in their net bag and place them perpendicular to the yoga block on the floor. The bottom ball should be touching the jaw muscle, whilst the top ball should be placed on the temple area during this exercise. Place your index finger on your cheek and trace the area where the bottom ball will go. Clench your teeth to find the muscle that pops up under your fingers- this is where you'll place the bottom ball. Lie down on your side with both knees bent, then slowly lower your head while still pinching the bottom ball between them until it rests in the traced area. Adjusting your yoga block may be necessary to ensure that pressure is being applied correctly bythe bottom ball- do so until you are comfortable. Having bent knees rather than straight legs will provide more stability for this exercise. You can twist your torso so that your chest is closer to the ground, and this movement will increase the pressure on the targeted area. Place one arm behind the yoga block while bending the other arm to support your position on the floor; there is no need to use additional force by pressing your head against ball as gravity will do that naturally. Remember breathe and relax your shoulder throughoutthe entire pose.

" Take long breaths by shifting your head up and down as you massage the top ball over your temples.

This should provide a full face massage to relieve neck tension and headaches. Let go of your jaw and open your mouth. You may stay in this posture for several minutes before repeating the process on the other side.

II. This exercise will focus on the neck, but the same equipment is required. This time, twist the therapeutic balls vertically. Place your index finger behind your ear and trace the spot where the ball takes it. There should be a bony bump here that you can feel with your finger; this is where you should place the back ball. Relax your shoulder and let your outer arm rest on top of your yoga block while keeping your inner arm parallel to it. For this exercise, you can also move your head. When you feel like you have spent enough time in this position, you can move your head facing sideways and place your chewing muscle on the top ball. To begin, find a comfortable position where you can tilt your head back and forth until you identify a sensitive spot. It should feel as though the massage is relieving tension in your jaw. After a few minutes, switch sides and repeat the process. To get out of this position, use both arms to lift yourself up from the yoga block and balls supporting your head - discard these once you're done. You should feel calm andnotice that muscle tension has dissipated on either side of the jawbone/mandible joint."

III. Sit down on a table with one therapeutic yoga ball. Rest one arm up and across your elbow. Grab the ball and position it at your temple. With your weight as pressure, lay your head to one side. If you feel that is too much pressure, lift your head higher if possible. You may apply as much force as you want by raising your head if it feels overly heavy. To massage your head with a ball, start by holding the ball between your palm and securing it to your head. Then, slide the ball back and forth across a larger area of your head. You can also massage your temples in circular motions as you breathe evenly throughout this technique. While placing the ball beneath your jaw on your neck, make sure to keep it level with your palm and continue sliding it back and forth. For more pressure, tilt your head side to side. Once you're in this position, slide the ball horizontally along the neck muscle towards behind your ears. Nod your head as if signaling yes and no as you hold the ball against your neck. Lastly, take the ball where the jaw meets. Place your head against the ball and open and close your mouth as you breathe in and out. The ball may also be rolled down and up in this region. You may circle the ball right in that area, to feel as though one exercise is better than the rest.

These exercises should take around 5 minutes on each side.

Repeat with the other side.

Foot Massage

Foot Massage activates the acupressure points imprinted on the foot's vagus nerve reflexes, which increases vagal activity. The release of oxytocin is triggered by an activated vagus nerve, and this hormone promotes relaxation, good digestion, and a sense of well-being. When massage is applied to the foot, the vagus nerve is stimulated, which then travels throughout the body and activates all of its organs for a feeling of being in excellent shape.

Even a gentle foot massage may assist in the re-balancing of the vagus nerve, lowering blood pressure. Vagus nerve stimulation is frequently used to help cancer patients cope with their stress and anxiety. Reflexology treatments can be combined.

The advantages of a chemical peel are typically apparent after just one treatment, but the effects of a long series of treatments, especially for someone with a long-term illness, may be even more dramatic.

Reflexology foot mat

The art of reflexology is pressure therapy that derives its origins from the belief different organs in our bodies correspond with certain areas of our feet. By using a foot chart as a guide, therapists can apply pressure to strategic points on their patient's feet; aiding in relaxation and healing throughout the body.

If you are seeking a natural and low-risk method to de-stress and unwind, reflexology may be right for you. Reflexology is often combined with other hands-on therapies, such as massage. In several trials, reflexology has been shown not only to alleviate pain but also psychological symptoms like tension and anxiety. Furthermore, it can help improve relaxation and sleep quality.

A reflexology foot mat may be found online and has two feet etched on it. The foot mat is made of high-quality rubber and includes approximately 1670 tiny cones, as well as a central instep hump. Its innovative design and special structure massage several important nerve endings in the soles of the feet. Using your body weight in conjunction with your Foot Massage Mat, you can stimulate all body parts, glands, and organs.

The Mat not only helps reduce stress but also improves the body's natural functioning. This, in turn, aids in maintaining good health for people of all ages. Some choose a rubber non-slip model that can be used in the shower. Although reflexology foot mats are more beneficial because of the cones, they're not suitable for shower use.

Sensory Deprivation tank

People are busier than ever, with home, employment, and self-care all competing for their attention. You're constantly jetting from one thing to the next, and even little things like going to the gym or performing hot yoga can be tiring. The sensory deprivation tank is a one-of-a-kind form of self-care.

Now, sensory deprivation may appear frightening, and sensory deprivation tanks might perhaps bring to mind images of science fiction, but the fact is that sensory deprivation tanks provide the ideal environment for tranquil encounters. You float in a warm, saline solution that keeps you effortlessly afloat.

When you enter a float tank, the water is warmed to match your body temperature. With deprived senses of sight, sound, and touch, it's an opportunity to have some well-deserved rest. You can find these tanks at health spas or wellness centers--they're often advertised as part of a self-care plan that also includes visits to saunas and massages.

You'll sit in the tank like a bathtub, then relax and float in the water, which will be about the same temperature as your skin. The tanks' water is often shallow; it's only 10 inches deep but contains approximately 800 pounds of salt, allowing you to float freely near the surface even if you fall asleep.

As you float calmly in the warm water, you have the option to turn off the lights and enjoy complete darkness and silence, or keep them on if that's more your speed. And if you're worried about being too cut-off from the world, don't fret—you can always choose to have soft music playing in the background.

There are three primary types of floating that are often used.

I. The primary pool is a larger, heated open-air pool that may accommodate one or two people. This is an excellent choice for claustrophobic individuals since the pools are not covered and are merely in a tiny space with no light or sound. These pools, however, owing to the fact that controlling light and sound in a wider space is more difficult, can't provide the most complete sensory deprivation experience.

II. An alternative to this is an afloat room, which gives you the chance to move around more freely but it does confine you within a five-by-eight area with an eight foot ceiling. You shouldn't worry too much about feeling enclosed because of how tall the ceiling is.

III. The final option is to float in a tank or pod. These look like large covered bathtubs. There is enough room inside for people to move around and sit up until the hatch is closed. Then, they are enclosed in the darkness and silence of the pod. This may be precisely what you need or it might be too much, depending on how you interact with space.

Floats typically last an hour, but some operators offer shorter or longer experiences. For example, some centers have floats that last up to seven hours! The SNS is activated during a float, which can cause increased heart rate, blood pressure, and other stress-related physical symptoms. Prior to the modern world,, such activation of the SNS was rare; now it happens virtually every day.

One approach to counteract the sympathetic nervous system's activity is to relax. Being calm is the polar opposite of being in fight or flight mode. As a consequence, slowing the sympathetic nervous system and increasing parasympathetic nerve activity reduces blood pressure and restarts the vagus nerve, which helps reduce anxiety.

Floating relieves a person's brain of a lot of stress, allowing them to talk with their feelings. Two physiological advantages of floating are lower blood pressure and slower heart rates. The physical benefits of floating, however, aren't limited to that.

Floating has been shown to help manage pain in certain studies. Floating in a sensory deprivation tank can help people with fibromyalgia and other chronic pain issues, according to studies. The muscles are relieved of all tension because the tank's environment replicates zero gravity. Furthermore, while floating activates the parasympathetic nervous system, it may aid in the healing process as well as relieve discomfort.

Give floating a chance! You could use some more relaxation in your life- be it physical or emotional. Listening to yourself think while floating might provide the fresh perspective you need to reach your goals when you're done, dried off, and ready to take action again. It's best practice to scope out the location before committing paying for your first session at a spa that offers this service.

Treating the Vagus Nerve

The vagus nerve is essential for the mind-body connection. Signals from the gut and organs that travel through the vagus nerve influence the entire brain. These messages affect emotions, and subconscious decisions are made from these signals that can greatly affect behavior.

The techniques to calculate exactly how the vagus nerve works are by assessing your heart rate variability. Your heart rate irregularities refer to any fluctuations that happen when you breathe.

Heart rate variability is associated with a greater capacity to recover from difficult circumstances. In contrast, decreased heart rate variability is linked to emotional detachment, stress, and anxiety that persists after a stressful event has passed.

The vagus nerve is a powerful tool that can help you regulate your heart rate and build resilience within your autonomic nervous system.

If you think of a recent stressful event, you might ask yourself:

- Just how long did it take for me to go back to a state of calm after I was stressed?

- Did the quantity of fear, anxiety, stress, and anger that came up for me appropriately match this scenario?

- Do I usually experience a feeling of worry or perhaps fear, although I know things are OK rationally?

- Do I get gastrointestinal issues after stress?

- Do I experience insomnia in difficult times?

Your physical health is linked to your mental well-being. Your mental states have a flow-on effect on your immune system, digestive system, lungs and heart, sleep, and social connection. Emotional problems can accelerate the aging process.

Not only will utilizing tools to balance your nervous system through the vagus nerve improve your long-term health (including immunity and digestion), but it will also help you foster deeper relationships.

With time and the right equipment, it's possible to transition from feeling anxious or afraid to feeling calm and at ease. The vagus nerve is responsible for relieving depression and anxiety, gastrointestinal issues, chronic pain, and sleep disturbances.

The neurological system under strain and dampen the inflammatory action with transcutaneous vagus nerve stimulation, acupuncture, and mind-body neural techniques. The markers of inflammation are altered by vagus nerve stimulation or increasing vagal tone.

The acupuncture points in the suboccipital auricular, which are near the nerve distribution area, activate the vagus nerve. The suboccipital auricular acupuncture points influence the vagus nerve. Acupuncture techniques that stimulate the vagus nerve are non-invasive, risk-free, and have no undesirable side effects.

The vagus nerve is the longest in our body, connecting the brain with many organs like the intestines, stomach, heart, and lungs. The vagus nerve is an important component of the "rest and digest" nervous system. It influences your breathing, digestive function, and heart rate - all of which have an impact on your mental health.

Furthermore, you need to be attentive to the sound of your vagus nerve. The vagus nerve is responsible for a number of activities in the body and its tone can influence how quickly we recover from stressors. A higher vagal tone indicates that we are more likely to relax when under duress.

Low vagal tone has been linked to poorer mental and attentional regulation, depression, and inflammation. This means the vagus nerve plays a crucial role in our body by being connected with conditions like anxiety. Although thisvagal tone is linked to immunity, emotional regulation, and metabolism, it can affect your stress sensitivity.

Vagus Nerve Treatment Through Acupuncture

Acupuncture has been used to treat a variety of ailments for more than 2,000 years. Acupuncture is a medical treatment in which small needles are inserted into designated body regions known as acupuncture points or perhaps acupoints.

Acupuncture is a type of healing that originated in Asia, and it is said to help Qi (pronounced "chee") flow throughout our bodies in the form of meridians. According to all those who use it, acupuncture inhibits or promotes Qi circulation according to need. Pathophysiological relationships between acupoints reflect the state of general health and abdominal organs. This is why specific acupoint stmulation may elicit a response from the vagus nerve and improve its tone.

Acupuncture stimulation is targeting the muscles by applying pressure to acupuncture points or areas closely related to them. However, with distal acupuncture stimulation, we are aiming for diseases that exist in internal organs; an example of this would be the vagus nerve.

Manual acupuncture is a type of Chinese medicine that uses a metallic needle to penetrate the skin and move it in one or both directions, thrusting and lifting. According to experts, patients may experience a tingly sensation that spreads throughout their bodies, which can be used to assess the therapeutic effectiveness of acupuncture. Based on testimonials, acupuncture is effective for many illnesses because of its ability to regulate inflammatory responses.

Treating the Vagus Nerve Through Mind-Body Therapy

A healthy vagus nerve is capable of comfortably supporting your digestive system, which aids in the regulation of sleep cycles and the relaxing of nerves. In individuals suffering from chronic illness, auto-immune disorders, migraines, vagus nerve anxiety, and depression, learning to regulate vagal tone is linked to decreased inflammation and a better prognosis.

The ventral vagal complex (VVC) will be the interpersonal communication system in soothing and calming. The term "social nervous system" comes from the fact that it controls facial expression.

Vagal Tone and Heart Rate Variability

The vagus nerve's good tone can be determined by the heart rate variability, or HRV, which are the oscillations in heart rate that happen when we breathe. To put it simply, there should minimal rise in heart rate upon inhaling and a decrease in heart rate when exhaling.

A healthy vagal tone is a balance of parasympathetic and sympathetic nervous system functions. Individuals with greater HRV can better transition from excitement to relaxation and recover more quickly from stress, in general.

Vagus Nerve Toning

Mind-body therapies, according to experts, relax and calm the mind while "safe mobilization and safe immobilization" of the body enhance resilience via the vagus nerve. This can help you feel more connected, peaceful, and tranquil in the beginning. You may gradually increase your tolerance for physiological reactivity as long as you have a solid basis for accessing your social central nervous system.

Your thoughts, emotional encounters, breath, and bodily sensations will also be addressed during this session. Furthermore, while Jessica's mind-body therapy is effective in treating your ideas and emotions as well as your breathing and physical symptoms, you may focus on perceiving the external world to determine your safety right now.

Conclusion

The complicated process that allows the mind and gut to interact with one another includes neural and endocrine links, as well as immunity and humoral communication.

The vagus nerve is crucial for the communication between the brain and gut. It plays a key role in inflammation, intestinal health, and hunger/fullness signals. We know that the vagus nerve affects what we eat, and how much of it we eat, which can impact weight gain.

Furthermore, the vagus nerve is crucial for regulating many functions in the body, including digestion, heart rate, and blood pressure. Vagus nerve stimulation has been shown to be beneficial for treating psychiatric disorders, obesity, and other stress-induced diseases.

When used with VNS, therapy is far more effective than VNS alone. When compared to extinction-only therapy, the combination of VNS and extinction is significantly more efficient. Because the FDA has granted it approval for treatment of depression and seizure prevention, VNS is an appealing and readily accessible addition to exposure therapy for treating severe anxiety disorders.

Vagus nerve stimulation has been shown to be an effective anticonvulsant device, and observational studies have indicated that it may also help reduce symptoms of depression. Because the vagus nerve sends information to brain regions necessary for the stress response, this pathway may be involved in sensing and manifesting various somatic and cognitive symptoms that characterize stress-related disorders.

Psychotropic drugs, like serotonin reuptake inhibitors, affect both the mind and the gastrointestinal tract and, consequently, should be known as modulators of the brain-gut axis.

Research that looks at the interactions between different nutrients, physical factors like heart rate, and psychological treatments has the potential to result in integrative treatment options. These could include VNS (vagal nerve stimulation), nutritional approaches, drugs, and psychological interventions like mindfulness-based approaches. The individual needs of each patient would be taken into account when customizing this type of treatment plan.

The vagus nerve, in collaboration with the nervous system, innervates the abdominal area. The nerve is responsible for sexual arousal because it extends to all the sexual parts. The nerve sends signals that start ovulation and other sexual activities.

When damage occurs to the nerve, there is a higher likelihood that abdominal pain will be experienced, especially by women.

www.ingramcontent.com/pod-product-compliance
Lightning Source LLC
Chambersburg PA
CBHW050358120526
44590CB00015B/1744